Presenting Your Case

Clifford D. Packer

Presenting Your Case

A Concise Guide for Medical Students

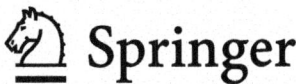 Springer

Clifford D. Packer, MD
Professor of Medicine
Department of Medicine
Case Western Reserve University School of Medicine
Louis Stokes Cleveland VA Medical Center
Cleveland, OH, USA

ISBN 978-3-030-13791-5   ISBN 978-3-030-13792-2   (eBook)
https://doi.org/10.1007/978-3-030-13792-2

Library of Congress Control Number: 2019935492

This Springer imprint is published by the registered company Springer
Nature Switzerland AG
The registered company address is: Gewerbestrasse 11, 6330 Cham, Switzerland

To my parents:
Sam Packer, MD (1915–2007)
Virginia Owen Packer, MD
(1924–2017)

Preface

In my 19 years as an internal medicine clerkship director, I have come to believe that the oral case presentation is a true rite of passage for third-year medical students. The ability to deliver a concise and thoughtful oral presentation is an important step in the transition from preclinical medicine to the art of medical practice. Unfortunately, learning to present well can be a difficult proposition. First, every attending seems to have slightly different expectations of what should be included in the oral presentation and how it should be organized. Second, the student must master a variety of presentation styles and formats; for example, transfer patients are presented differently than direct admissions, and presentations are structured differently on the wards, in the emergency room, and in the outpatient clinic. Third, it has been shown that medical students tend to view their role as passive presenters of facts and data, whereas attendings and residents expect a robust discussion of the differential diagnosis and treatment plan.

Students who master the oral presentation quickly are accepted as full team members and given additional privileges and responsibilities; students who struggle are sometimes viewed as disorganized and lacking in medical knowledge. The strugglers worry about their clerkship grade and how it might affect their residency options, which produces more performance anxiety and more confusion. I have seen students literally writhing with anxiety as they present their patients. This should never happen.

I wrote this book to demystify and deconstruct the oral case presentation, with the simple goal of increasing third-year students' confidence and reducing their anxiety as they step up to present their first patients on the wards. I was inspired by the words of Rachel K. Sobel, who truly understands the importance of the oral presentation and has this wise counsel for students:

> Fluency always takes time. With more experience, the oral presentation will no longer feel like a structured exercise in data collection, with an exhaustive list of blanks to fill in and a write-up as cue-card. Presenting, in time, will become the beginning of a beautiful conversation.

This "beautiful conversation" is a perfect aspirational definition of the oral case presentation. It is not meant to be a one-sided recital; it is more than just a list of facts and figures that anyone can access in the electronic medical record. At some point, it should become an exchange of ideas in conversational form. It should be about teaching, learning, and discussing patient management, not checklists and rigid presenting scripts. "Just tell us the story," attendings should say to their students on the first day of the clerkship, "and then tell us what you think."

Readers of this book will soon realize that my approach to the oral case presentation and related topics is empirical, based mainly on my experience as a clerkship director. The reason for this is that I am constitutionally unable to read even the most brilliant articles on educational theory. However, I have included a few simple theoretical frameworks, such as SNAPPS and SOAP-V, which are practical, useful, and easy for students to implement in their case presentations. The rest is a mixture of actual, composite, and invented student case presentations, along with a few (hopefully not irrelevant) digressions on such topics as differential diagnosis, pimping, high-value care, and the effects of new technologies on the case presentation.

I would like to thank several people for their help with this book. Dr. Thomas Hornick, my friend and VA colleague, kindly read several chapters of the manuscript and gave me helpful comments and encouragement. Dr. Jeffrey Krimmel-Morrison, now a rising chief resident at the University of Washington, graciously allowed me to use his insightful comments on decisiveness from an email he sent me as a medical student (see Chap. 11; his views have changed dramatically since then!). Diane Lamsback, my terrific developmental editor at Springer, helped enormously with the figures and permissions and kept me on track to finish the book on schedule. Finally, I would like to thank my wife, Marie, who took my 10 months of evenings and weekends at the computer in stride, for her enduring patience and support.

Cleveland, OH, USA   Clifford D. Packer, MD, FACP
December 30, 2018

Contents

Chapter 1
The Importance of a Good Case Presentation and Why Students Struggle with It

Morning Rounds

It's a busy morning on the wards. There were several new patients admitted overnight, and the team is at full capacity. The attending physician arrives, greets the team, and takes a quick look at the new names on the board. "Everybody stable?" he asks, and the senior resident nods her head. "OK then, let's get going."

The senior resident leads the way to the first new patient, an elderly man who came in late last night with shortness of breath. The third-year medical student pulls out a sheaf of papers and begins to read: "The patient is an 83-year-old man who presented with shortness of breath. He also had some sharp chest pain and a new rash on the back of his neck that's very itchy. I think it's a fungal rash. He's also had some worsening back pain lately, but that's more of a chronic thing. His straight leg raise was negative, I think – I'm not sure I was doing it right. But the main thing is this shortness of breath. He says he's not wheezing, but when I listened to his lungs I thought I might have heard some expiratory wheezes. He's also coughing up some yellow phlegm, but he didn't have any rales or egophony. I don't think he has pneumonia. He didn't have a fever. His ankles have been a little swollen. He also gets heartburn about twice a week lately."

© Springer Nature Switzerland AG 2019
C. D. Packer, *Presenting Your Case*,
https://doi.org/10.1007/978-3-030-13792-2_1

"What about his hospitalization for heart failure 2 weeks ago?" the intern interjects helpfully.

"I was saving that for the past medical history," says the student. "He has hypertension, type 2 diabetes, heart failure with preserved ejection fraction, aortic stenosis, gout, low back pain, an inguinal hernia, and a pilonidal cyst. He was hospitalized for heart failure at an outside hospital 2 weeks ago. I couldn't get the records overnight. They gave him Lasix and he lost 20 pounds."

"But he had gained back 15 pounds as of last night," adds the intern. "And he has three pillow orthopnea, PND, and worsening leg edema."

"I forgot to mention that," says the student. "On review of systems, he's been having black stools for a while. He takes ibuprofen 800 mg three times a day, sometimes more, for his back pain. He also thinks he might have had a gout flare in his left wrist about 3 weeks ago. And he gets tension head-aches about three times a week."

"One other thing," adds the intern. "His hemoglobin has dropped from 12.3 a month ago to 6.2 on admission last night."

"That's right," says the student, "and he had a little epigas-tric tenderness and maybe some rebound on his abdominal exam. I wasn't sure about my technique. But I did hear active bowel sounds."

Of course, even an attending with the patience of Job would have interrupted this meandering, disorganized pre-sentation several times by now. When did the shortness of breath begin? Did it progress and limit his activity? Any recent travel, surgery, or immobilization? Any smoking his-tory? Was the sharp chest pain pleuritic? Was it substernal, exertional, relieved with rest or nitroglycerin? Was there any associated dyspnea, nausea, or diaphoresis? What else do we know about his recent hospitalization and his heart failure history? What is his aortic valve area? Was he orthostatic on admission? How long has the melena been going on? Any history of upper or lower GI bleeding, or iron deficiency ane-mia? Any recent endoscopies? And what about the vital signs and the rest of the physical exam?

What are the problems with this student's oral case presentation? The timeline – the most important component of the history of present illness (HPI) – is confusing and incomplete. The overall organization is chaotic. The editing is poor, with several important omissions and an inappropriate focus on trivial details. Important symptoms are poorly and incompletely described. The narrative skips frequently from subjective to objective to assessment, with bouts of uncertainty and self-criticism that reflect the student's lack of confidence. At this point, the attending will probably turn to the intern to get the full story. The intern fills in the important points from the H&P, and the thoughtful senior resident hypothesizes that the patient now has high-output heart failure due to a subacute NSAID-induced upper GI bleed, possibly aggravated by aortic stenosis. The student is out of the loop.

This is not a "real" case presentation but rather a composite of the many weak oral presentations I have heard in my 21 years as a VA ward attending. Many students, even brilliant ones, tend to overthink and overanalyze their presentations, defending and explaining every finding they present, going off on tangents, and finally petering out without a clear path to the diagnosis. They fail to realize that the case presentation should be a straightforward narrative of the patient's history and objective findings, structured as a timeline, and leading logically to a diagnosis. The case presentation, in other words, is where the student tells the story and makes an argument for what they think is ailing the patient. It is not meant to be (or not to be) a Hamlet-like soliloquy of self-doubt and metaphysical uncertainty. It is a structured recitation of the facts that leads to a well-supported argument.

Meanwhile, what has been happening on morning rounds? The day is off to a slow start. Much backtracking was needed to get the full story of the first new patient. The student is not quite sure what went wrong with his case presentation. He wonders if he should ask for feedback. As rounds continue, several complex patients are seen, and their management plans are discussed. The student tries to follow the discussion but grows more distracted and withdrawn as he continues to mull over his abortive case presentation. He wants to go into internal medicine and become a cardiologist, but he is beginning to worry about his clerkship grade.

Why Students Struggle

The paradoxical nature of the oral presentation is reflected in the way a good presentation is described: *thorough yet concise; focused but sufficiently comprehensive; included all pertinent positives and negatives; the initial differential diagnosis was broad; and then it was narrowed appropriately.* The cognitive challenge of the oral presentation is its mix of exposition and argument: the speaker is simultaneously giving a concise description of the case and – by the way the description is focused and edited – an argument for a particular diagnosis. This requires a strong knowledge base and a method for differential diagnosis. New students generally have a good knowledge of basic science but are lacking in clinical knowledge and differential diagnosis skills. They are trained as data gatherers. The function of the clerkship is to begin the process of turning these data gatherers into astute clinical thinkers. The oral case presentation is a bellwether for this crucial transition. Students who have mastered the case presentation are recognized as ready to contribute and take on additional responsibility.

Oral case presentations can be very stressful for medical students. The case presentation is a solo performance given for an impatient and potentially hostile audience. Stage fright can lead to confusion and disorganization. Attendings and residents interrupt frequently; an observational study of medical trainees' oral case presentations in the emergency room found that interruptions occurred at a rate of 0.75 per minute, with an average of 2.49 interruptions per presentation [1]. Even well-organized students can become flustered when they are repeatedly interrupted to answer questions or expand on their findings.

But beyond performance stress, the biggest reason students struggle is that they are unprepared. "Case presentation, so universally required, is poorly taught," commented Kurt Kroenke in 1985 [2], and little seems to have changed since then. In my 18 years as a medicine clerkship director, I have observed that the student who is prepared to give a concise and organized oral presentation in the first week of the clerkship is as rare as hen's teeth. Although all students know the basic structure and order of presentation – the chief complaint, HPI, past medical and surgical history, medications, allergies, family history, social history, review of systems, physical exam, lab and imaging results, assessment, and plan – they do not know how to prioritize, edit, and focus their data. Students feel a tremendous pressure to describe *everything* they have learned about the patient – every detail of the history, every physical finding – and it comes pouring out, often in no particular order and with little thought about the relevance of the finding. In his wonderful essay on case presentation [2], Kroenke writes that "an artful presentation contains the right facts in the proper order selectively emphasized." He describes the peregrination (wandering) from place to place and the preoccupation with equal time for all findings that bedevil student presentations. "Effective presentations are not so democratic" he continues:

> ...Present what is relevant. Do not recite verbatim the fine print of your write-up. Avoid prolix descriptions of retinal arteries or integument. Spare your listeners euglycemia, P-R intervals, and the 20 values of a chemistry profile. Focus on findings that were abnormal or, if normal, related to active problems. Regarding the remainder of the findings, a simple statement that they were normal is sufficient. [2]

Students learn these lessons on the wards, gradually and sometimes painfully, and most are presenting their patients reasonably well by the end of their medicine clerkships. The problem is that some students progress very slowly with their presentations and come to be perceived by their evaluators as disorganized or lacking in medical knowledge. Since attending physicians do not necessarily observe students as they perform H&Ps and provide direct patient care [3], the oral case presentation is often the primary basis for grading a student's clinical performance. Students are aware of this, understand that the stakes are high, and put an enormous amount of time and energy into their case presentations. For students who are slow to grasp the correct form and function of the oral presentation, this can lead to excessively long and angst-ridden performances that are then picked apart by the attending on rounds. At this point, most students ask for guidance and eventually are able to focus and streamline their presentations. The process usually takes several weeks. Table 1.1 gives my current medicine clerkship students' responses when they were asked to identify areas of self-improvement in their mid-rotation assessment. All students

TABLE 1.1 "Based on your self-assessment and feedback, identify one or more areas you want to work on to improve during the remainder of the rotation" (From mid-rotation student self-assessments, January–March 2018)

I have been working on improving my presentation organization and wording. I've got the general order down but sometimes could communicate things more clearly and focus on pertinent details. Originally, I worked on being complete with my presentations, but recently I've received feedback that I should focus on the more acute/active issues instead of listing out every detail. I would also like to continue improving in my assessment/planning abilities

My presentations are too long and I will work to shorten them

I am still working on oral presentations and presenting things in an organized way

One area that I would like to improve on during the remainder of the rotation is developing the assessment in my oral presentations

I would like to improve on my presentations

I would like to continue working on my assessment, plan, and differential. I am currently trying to parse my presentations down to pertinent positives and negatives, as well as improve my assessment/plan for to include all of the patient's problems that need to be managed during a hospital stay were 3–4 weeks into their 6-week inpatient rotation when these comments were collected. Clearly, the oral presentation is an ongoing concern for many students even as they head into the home stretch of the clerkship.

One might argue that this is a normal rite of passage and that the struggle to master the oral presentation leaves no long-term scars. Perhaps, but why teach this important skill in such a random and scattershot way? Why do our students understand the subtleties of acid-base physiology and the Starling curve but struggle needlessly with putting together an effective case presentation? The purpose of this book is to explain and demystify the student case presentation and ease the difficult transition from the classroom to the hospital. Chapters 2, 3, 4, 5, 6, and 7 describe the various types of oral presentations and their organization, the importance of the timeline in the HPI, how to focus and edit the presentation, and how to create a robust assessment and an actionable plan. Chapter 8 gives a detailed and practical approach to differential diagnosis. Chapter 9 describes how to cite the literature effectively in an oral presentation. Chapter 10 explains how to add a discussion of high value care – including costs of care – using a simple and innovative method called SOAP-V. Chapter 11 expounds on how to get involved in rounds and participate in care discussions and decision-making. Chapter 12 takes aim at the notorious problem of "pimping," the aggressive and sometimes unfair questioning that can be directed at students on rounds. Chapter 13 describes how to prepare and deliver a useful and engaging 5-minute talk. Finally, Chap. 14 explores the effects of technology and cultural change on the future of the case presentation.

As you read this book, the key point to understand is that the same traits that will make you an outstanding physician – intelligence, compassion, humanism, persistence, integrity, and creativity – will also bring success and fulfillment in your clerkships. Walter Pater, the English essayist and art critic, wrote: "To burn always with this hard, gem-like flame, to maintain this ecstasy, is success in life [4]." The guidance and advice offered in this book may help, but there are no substitutes for passion and idealism in the life of a physician. Speak up on rounds, engage in discussion, and satisfy your curiosity by reading and asking questions. Stand up for your patients: treat their pain and anxiety, make sure they understand what is happening, and ask them about their own goals of care. Use your intelligence, think creatively, and advocate for an experimental treatment or a new approach if you think it will help. Present your case well, and others will listen.

References

1. Yang G, Chin R. Assessment of teacher interruptions on learners during oral case presentations. Acad Emerg Med. 2007;14(6):521–5.
2. Kroenke K. The case presentation. Stumbling blocks and stepping stones. Am J Med. 1985;79(5):605–8.
3. Schiller J, Hammoud M, Belmonte D, Englesbe M, Gelb D, Grum C, et al. Systematic direct observation of clinical skills in the clinical year. MedEdPORTAL. 2014;10:9712.
4. Pater W. Studies in the history of the renaissance. New York: Oxford University Press; 2010.

Chapter 2
Organization of the Oral Case Presentation

Medicine is a science of uncertainty and an art of probability.
William Osler

The Admission H&P Versus the Oral Case Presentation

When presenting a new patient on the wards, medical students often assume that the best approach is simply to read their full history and physical to the team on rounds. They see the oral presentation as a rigid, rule-based recitation of clinical data, while their teachers view it as a flexible means of communication that uses the data to construct a diagnosis and treatment plan [1]. As the student reads, the intern sighs and starts tapping on his phone, the resident turns away to enter orders in the computer, and the attending, after listening politely for a minute or two, launches a fusillade of questions meant to cut to the chase and get the essential information needed to make a diagnosis and set up a plan of care for the patient. The student, who spent 2 hours with the patient and worked very hard on her H&P, feels upset because she has been denied the opportunity to show her thoroughness. The presentation, rather than flowing from the student, is extracted by the attending.

This is a common scenario, especially in the early days of the clerkship. The student has not yet learned that the oral

© Springer Nature Switzerland AG 2019
C. D. Packer, *Presenting Your Case*,
https://doi.org/10.1007/978-3-030-13792-2_2

case presentation differs from the admission H&P in scope, structure, and function. The admission H&P is a meticulous and detailed written report of the patient's history, complete physical exam, allergies, medications, family history, social history, and review of systems. It serves as an important archive of baseline information on the new patient, to which any caregiver can refer. The oral presentation, on the other hand, is a focused and carefully edited production that both gives the essential clinical information and builds the argument for a particular diagnosis. It includes a concise and focused summary of the H&P, followed by a discussion of the differential diagnosis and a plan of action. It is not meant to be all-inclusive and archival; it is essentially an argument, a hypothesis based on the facts of the case. It is meant to persuade as well as inform the listener. Another way to think of it is as a thesis that is presented and then defended by the student. It is active, fluid, and discussable.

The SOAPS Method [2] is a useful way to understand and approach the oral case presentation. The authors surveyed North American clerkship directors and clinician-teachers on the most valuable content for the oral case presentation (OCP) of a new patient by third-year medical students. From the survey data, they developed a structured approach to teaching and evaluating the OCP. They identified five core qualities of an effective OCP:

- **Story**: The OCP describes key clinical facts.
- **Organization**: The facts are where the listener expects.
- **Argument**: The OCP makes the case for assessment and plan.
- **Pertinence**: The OCP includes only information relevant to the assessment and plan.
- **Speech**: The OCP is articulate.

The authors further describe the elements of the SOAPS oral presentation:

- **Story** *means weaving the "facts" into a coherent narrative summary. The story is a chronological description of the manifestations of illness, attempted interventions, and patient interpretations. The learner fully characterizes the* *most prominent symptoms. The story includes the context in which these symptoms occur, including baseline functional status and relevant elements from past medical history, social history,* etc.

- **Organization** *relates to the OCP's use as a tool to transfer patient care information among providers. Providing facts when listeners expect them allows listeners to easily absorb the material. Thus, following common "standards" of presentation, such as presenting history before physical, is essential. Equally important is the logical organization of facts, such as grouping symptoms by possible diagnoses (rather than organ systems).*

- **Argument.** *The presentation makes an argument for a diagnosis (or limited differential) or a plan. The learner commits to a specific diagnosis or a few possible diagnoses, and structures the OCP to support this thesis. The presentation should lead listeners to the expected conclusion. Note that although standard organization and pertinence are necessary to structure a good argument, a well-organized and pertinent presentation can still fail to make an argument.*

- **Pertinence** *relates to including only the important facts. For example, a series of negative blood cultures would be pertinent to an infectious disease consultant but not to the cardiology team managing unstable angina. "Pertinence" and "argument" are related, and it would be difficult to have a well-argued presentation that lacked pertinence. However, the converse is not true.*

- **Speech.** *While the first four qualities could be applied to written notes as well, "speech" recognizes that the OCP is an exercise in public speaking. The presentation should be free of repetition and "umms," spoken at an appropriate volume and speed. Since body language and eye contact are important, the presentation should not be read from notes.* [2][1]

As the American architect Louis Sullivan famously declared in 1910, "Form follows function." Since the oral

---

[1] Quoted with permission from the Alliance for Academic Internal Medicine.

presentation serves a different function than the admission H&P, its form must be different as well. Figure 2.1 presents a schema for the oral case presentation, which takes into account the SOAPS Method and shows how the various parts of the traditional H&P can be modified, condensed, or omitted in the oral presentation.

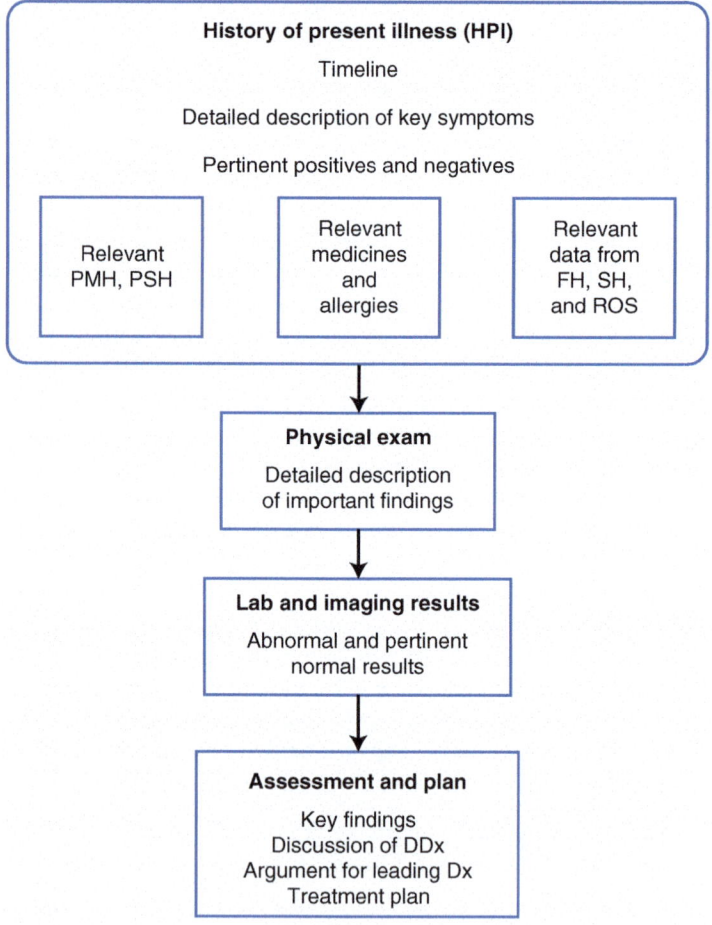

FIGURE 2.1 Schema of the oral case presentation

The History of Present Illness (HPI)

The HPI is the foundation of the oral case presentation. It tells the story, clarifies the sequence and relatedness of events, and builds the case for a possible diagnosis. It begins with the patient's age, gender, and major medical problems and continues with a timeline describing the clinical events:

> The patient is a 68-year-old woman with hypertension, type 2 diabetes mellitus, and hypothyroidism. She was in her usual state of health until 5 days before admission, when she developed dysuria and mild malaise. Three days before admission, she spiked a fever to 101 degrees and noted the onset of low back pain, worse on the left side. Yesterday, she developed nausea and vomiting and was unable to keep down fluids, so she went to the emergency room.

A timeline is essential to show temporal relationships that can be used to argue for cause and effect (as in adverse drug reactions) or the development of symptoms over time to indicate possible disease etiologies according to natural history (as with the onset of atypical versus bacterial pneumonia). Even in apparently simple cases, as above, the timeline gives a clear, linear description of the course of events. In a very sick patient with multiple serious problems and a complicated ICU course, an accurate timeline is even more important. Flow sheets of fever curves, sodium levels, platelet counts, and so forth can also be presented in the HPI to show relationships and help to argue for a diagnosis. For additional discussion of the HPI and examples of timelines and flow charts, see Chap. 4.

Another important feature of the HPI in an oral presentation is the sponge-like way it absorbs relevant information from the family history, social history, and review of systems. This allows for presentation of all relevant data in one place, so that it can be connected and remembered, rather than pieced together from scattered parts of the history. The HPI continues:

> She has a history of two urinary tract infections over the past 3 years; in both cases, urine cultures grew pan-sensitive *E.coli*, and treatment with oral trimethoprim-sulfamethoxazole was successful. Of note, she has a new male sexual partner and has had problems with vaginal dryness and dyspareunia. She has a younger

sister who had surgery for a congenital urinary tract disorder in childhood. She has no personal or family history of kidney stones. Since her last UTI 6 months ago, she has been taking a probiotic supplement that contains cranberry extract and D-mannose. She has chronic low back pain, but the pain associated with her recent illness is more intense and radiates to the left flank.

Note how pertinent data from the social history, family history, review of systems, and even the OTC medication list have been moved to the HPI in order to streamline the presentation. This reorganization helps both presenter and listener to think about the broad differential diagnosis and narrow it as more information becomes available. The symptoms and facts of the case are grouped according to a possible diagnosis (UTI, pyelonephritis) rather than by organ systems.

The HPI continues with pertinent positives and negatives and concludes with a brief description of her emergency room course, ending with the rationale for her hospital admission:

She has not noticed any vaginal discharge, hematuria, or urinary incontinence. She does have urinary frequency since the onset of symptoms. There is no chest pain, shortness of breath, cough, or abdominal pain. In the ER, she was febrile and orthostatic, and was given IV hydration with resolution of the orthostatic symptoms. Blood and urine cultures were taken, and she was started on IV ceftriaxone and admitted for urinary tract infection, rule out urosepsis.

(Some attendings prefer not to have the ER course included in the HPI. I prefer to hear it because the HPI is meant to tell the full story, from onset of illness to hospitalization. I want to know the reason for the decision to hospitalize the patient early on in the presentation, so I'm not left wondering about it.)

Past Medical History and Past Surgical History

The patient's significant medical problems – hypertension, type 2 diabetes, and hypothyroidism – were listed in the first line of the HPI. *They do not need to be repeated.* If she had poorly controlled diabetes or profound hypothyroidism, those issues should be discussed in the HPI. *Minor medical problems that have no bearing on the case do not need to be mentioned in the oral presentation.* As for past surgical history, a history of surgery for bladder prolapse or vesicovaginal fistula would be mentioned prominently in the HPI because it is potentially relevant to the presenting symptoms. Past surgeries for a wrist fracture, cataracts, or hammertoes are irrelevant and should not be mentioned in the oral presentation (although they must be listed for completeness in the written admission H&P).

Medications

While some attendings insist on a recitation of the full medication list, including eyedrops, nasal sprays, and topical creams, I think that list-reading can kill the momentum of a good oral presentation. Medicines that are immediately relevant to the presenting complaint should be mentioned in the HPI; otherwise, they can be discussed in the assessment and plan, when medication management is reviewed. In the above case, we would probably want to hold the patient's metformin and lisinopril because of her dehydration and risk for acute kidney injury.

Allergies

Allergies that may have a significant bearing on testing and treatment, such as penicillin or IV contrast allergies, should be mentioned in the HPI. Less significant drug allergies do not need to be mentioned in the oral presentation unless they are specifically connected to the presenting complaint or pose a potential problem with treatment.

Family History

As discussed above, any relevant family history should be taken up in the HPI. Significant but not directly relevant items, such as a strong family history of premature coronary artery disease, brain aneurysm, or colon cancer, can be noted briefly, especially if they raise screening or management issues that will need to be addressed.

Social History

As with the family history, relevant data from the social history (such as the patient's sexual history in the case described above) should be included in the HPI. One can argue, however, that the entire social history is relevant for every patient, given the importance of the social determinants of health and disease. Table 2.1 shows the important elements of the social history. As an attending, I like to hear the complete social history for all of my new patients, mainly because the

TABLE 2.1 Elements of the social history

Social history categories	Comments
Tobacco use	In pack-years; ask about smokeless tobacco
Alcohol use	In units of alcohol per day or week
Illicit drug use	Increased risk of hepatitis B/C and HIV with IV drug use
Family and marital status	Support system; divorce, separation, dependents
Sexual history	Sexual orientation; current sexual activity; use of condoms, other contraceptives
Living situation	Homelessness, foreclosure; inadequate or unsafe housing
Education level	Highest level or degree attained
Occupational history	Potential exposures, injuries, or other stressors
Military service history	Screen for PTSD, traumatic brain injury, military sexual trauma as indicated
Travel history	Travel to endemic areas

yield of useful information is so high. Knowing that this patient was homeless, or had untreated PTSD, or was functionally illiterate might lead to significant changes in the treatment and follow-up plan.

Review of Systems

The review of systems (ROS) is a comprehensive assessment of the patient's current health status. Its aim is to identify any important issues that were not revealed in the initial exploration of the presenting complaint. In general, for the oral presentation, any relevant or significant data from the ROS should be presented in the HPI. In the above case, the patient's chronic low back pain is relevant because back pain is also one of her presenting complaints; it is noted that "the pain associated with her recent illness is more intense and radiates to the left flank." Any other significant findings from the ROS, such as chest pain, shortness of breath, unilateral leg swelling, or a positive depression screen, should be mentioned and further discussed in the HPI. Trivial or unrelated ROS findings, such as chronic shoulder pain, eczema, pes planus, or mild constipation, are documented in the written H&P but should not be included in the oral presentation.

Physical Exam

In the oral presentation, it is important to show that a complete physical exam was performed, but attention should be focused on the relevant findings. *The time spent describing an exam finding should be proportional to its importance in the case.* A patient admitted with cellulitis and leg ulcers should have a detailed description of the location, size, color, and depth of the ulcers and the presence of granulation tissue, slough, or eschar; the extent of the cellulitis and the presence of fluctuance, bullae, or oozing should be carefully described. A patient with hepatomegaly and an abdominal mass should have a similarly meticulous description of the abdominal exam. This seems obvious, but many students give lavish descriptions of normal or inconsequential findings and then seem to run out of energy when it comes to describing the most important findings.

In general, a head-to-toe approach is the best way to organize the data and remember all of the key findings. Always begin with the complete vital signs, plus the current O_2 saturation including the FiO_2. To return to our patient with fever, back pain, and dysuria, the oral presentation now continues with the physical exam findings:

> On physical exam, the vital signs were temperature 101.7 degrees, pulse 92, respiratory rate 16, and blood pressure 105/67. The O2 saturation was 94% on room air. The oral mucosa was dry, and there was diminished skin turgor. There was no cervical lymphadenopathy or thyromegaly, and the jugular venous pressure was less than 5 cm. The lungs were clear to auscultation and percussion; the heart was regular, with an S4 gallop and no murmurs. Examination of the back revealed no lumbar spinous or paraspinous tenderness and no muscle spasm; straight leg raise was negative. There was marked CVA tenderness on the left side only. On abdominal exam, the bowel sounds were present but diminished; there was no abdominal distention; the liver span was normal by percussion, and the spleen was not palpable; there was mild left mid-abdominal tenderness to deep palpation, with no guarding or rebound tenderness. The extremities were warm, with 2+ DP and PT pulses in the feet bilaterally and no peripheral edema. Neurologic exam revealed normal mental status, normal cranial nerves II-XII, and globally normal motor, sensory, and cerebellar function.

Note that the most relevant parts of the exam – the abdomen, the back, and the assessment for volume status and signs of sepsis – are described in the greatest detail. Note also that the student has presented the physical findings firmly, with no indecision, vacillation, or superfluous explanation. It is fine for students to admit uncertainty about their physical exam skills and ask for help and confirmation. However, the report of the physical exam in an oral presentation should not become a series of half-baked observations interspersed with apologies. *Commit to your findings.* If you want confirmation, ask the attending to repeat the relevant parts of the exam with you at the bedside afterward.

Laboratory Tests and Imaging Results

In reporting the initial laboratory and imaging data, a good rule of thumb is that all significant abnormal results *and* pertinent normal results should be given. "Lab results were significant for…" is a good way to begin. The attending is immediately aware that the student has done some thinking about the test results and decided which were most relevant. This editing is part of the "argument for a diagnosis" thread that should run through the whole case presentation. The case presentation continues:

> Lab results were significant for a white blood cell count of 13,000 with 88% neutrophils; the sodium was 144, potassium 3.7, chloride 108, bicarb 24, BUN 32, and creatinine 1.4 (with a baseline of 0.9 3 months ago). The glucose was 127. The serum lipase was normal at 76. Urinalysis revealed 350 WBC's with positive nitrite and leukocyte esterase. Blood and urine culture results are pending. KUB revealed a non-specific bowel gas pattern with no evidence of ileus or obstruction, no bowel wall thickening, and no sign of kidney stones. Chest x-ray was normal.

In this case, the leukocytosis, pyuria, and prerenal azotemia are the most important abnormal lab findings. The unremarkable electrolyte and lipase results are also presented because they are pertinent normals in a patient admitted with nausea, vomiting, and dehydration. The KUB, which shows no evidence of kidney stones, bowel obstruction, ileus, or bowel ischemia, is particularly important in terms of narrowing the differential diagnosis. The chest x-ray is also useful in that there is no evidence of pneumonia in this elderly patient with fever. At this point, thanks to the student's focused and well-organized presentation, a likely diagnosis has clearly emerged.

The Assessment and Plan

The first step in making as assessment is to collect the key findings from the history, physical exam, and initial lab and imaging results. Collecting the key findings is a way to distil the case down to its basic elements in order to think about it, discuss it, and formulate a differential diagnosis. Table 2.2 lists the key findings in the case under discussion. In the assessment, start by organizing the key findings into a concise summary of the case:

> In summary, this is a 68-year-old woman with a history of type 2 diabetes and two prior UTIs who presented with dysuria, fever, nausea, vomiting, and acute back pain. Her physical exam was significant for fever to 101.7 degrees and left CVA tenderness. Initial testing revealed leukocytosis and pyuria; her KUB was negative.

The next step is to give a broad differential diagnosis, based again on the key findings and taking into account uncommon or atypical presentations that might mimic more common conditions:

> The differential diagnosis for a patient with fever and back or flank pain is broad, especially in an elderly patient, who is more likely to have an atypical clinical presentation for an intra-abdominal infection. The broad differential includes pyelonephritis, diverticulitis,

TABLE 2.2 Key findings in this case

From the history	From the physical exam	From lab/imaging results
Dysuria	Fever to 101.7	Leukocytosis
Fever	Left CVA tenderness	Pyuria
Nausea		Negative KUB
Vomiting		
Back pain		
Prior urinary tract infections		
Type 2 diabetes		

cholecystitis, appendicitis, nephrolithiasis with obstruction, colo-
vesical fistula, soft tissue infection, intra-abdominal abscess, and
lumbar discitis, osteomyelitis, or epidural abscess.

Finally, the differential diagnosis must be narrowed, with
an argument to support the likeliest diagnosis and reasons
that the competing diagnoses are less likely:

> I think that the most likely diagnosis in this case is pyelonephritis.
> The dysuria and pyuria suggest a urinary tract infection, and the
> 5-day course with high fever, leukocytosis, nausea and vomiting,
> flank pain, and unilateral CVA tenderness strongly supports the
> diagnosis of pyelonephritis. While other intra-abdominal infec-
> tions are possible, the location and radiation of the pain and the
> physical findings are not typical of cholecystitis, appendicitis, or
> diverticulitis. The absence of blood in the urine and radiopaque
> stones on KUB are against the presence of obstructing kidney
> stones. There was no pneumaturia, so a colovesical fistula is
> unlikely. Epidural abscess is very unlikely with CVA rather than
> spinous tenderness, and multiple findings that support the urinary
> tract as the source of infection.

A comment on the decision-making process in the context
of high-value care is sometimes appropriate, especially when
a commonly ordered test, treatment, or procedure would
increase cost but add little value (see Chap. 10):

> We considered ordering an abdominal CT, but decided that it
> would be unlikely to change our management, given the high
> probability of pyelonephritis based on all of the clinical data.

The treatment plan should cover major management
issues such as selection and dosing of medications, IV fluids,
transfusions, important nursing orders such as I/Os or neuro
checks, and treatment protocols such as CIWA for alcohol
withdrawal or APACHE for sepsis. The details of insulin sliding scales and minor dose adjustments of antihypertensive
drugs or diuretics usually do not need to be discussed in the
oral presentation. Our case continues:

> For the patient's dehydration and prerenal azotemia, we will con-
> tinue the IV normal saline at 150 cc/hr and hold her lisinopril and
> metformin until the creatinine has returned to baseline. For the
> pyelonephritis and possible urosepsis, we will continue IV ceftri-
> axone pending blood and urine culture results. When the culture

results are available, we'll narrow the antibiotic spectrum accordingly. Ceftriaxone should cover the likely gram-negative pathogens such as *E.coli* and *K. pneumoniae* with a very low probability of antibacterial resistance, according to our hospital antibiogram. No additional imaging is indicated at present, but if her fever persists beyond 48-72 hours on the ceftriaxone, we would have to consider abdominal CT or ultrasound to rule out perinephric abscess or obstruction.

Not included in this transcript of an oral case presentation are the comments, questions, and discussion points that are typically raised by the attending and senior resident. For medical students, there is an art to answering these questions while at the same time maintaining the organization and momentum of the case presentation. Preparation is crucial. *Rehearse the case presentation beforehand, without notes. Memorize the timeline and the key findings. Tell the story, and make an argument for the diagnosis. These are the best ways to prepare and deliver an effective oral presentation.*

References

1. Haber RJ, Lingard LA. Learning oral presentation skills: a rhetorical analysis with pedagogical and professional implications. J Gen Intern Med. 2001;16(5):308–14.
2. Green EH, Fagan MJ, Sharpe B, deCherrie L, Hershman W. Using a structured approach to teaching and evaluating oral case presentations: the SOAPS method. Acad Intern Med Insight. 2011;9(3):6–8.

Chapter 3
Variations on the Oral Case Presentation

Night Float Admissions

Ever since the adoption of strict work-hour requirements for interns and residents, night float admissions are common in teaching hospitals. Sometimes the night-admitting resident stays to present the patient on morning rounds, but more often the handoff occurs before rounds. Medical students who are assigned to these patients may end up simply reading the admitting resident's full history and physical, with its already-formulated assessment and plan, to the team. The educational value of such a presentation is practically nil.

A more active approach to the night float presentation can provide a higher-quality educational experience for the student, a more vigorous discussion of the case, and – arguably – better care for the patient. On busy nights, when many patients are admitted, the night float resident focuses on ruling out life-threatening problems, making a provisional diagnosis, and initiating a reasonable course of treatment. In the morning, a respectful critique of the resident's initial assessment is essential. Anything can happen overnight and often does. The treatment plan might need a few tweaks, or the whole trajectory of the case might need to be reevaluated.

First, the student should see and examine the patient before morning rounds, if possible, and collect the latest

© Springer Nature Switzerland AG 2019
C. D. Packer, *Presenting Your Case*,
https://doi.org/10.1007/978-3-030-13792-2_3

clinical, lab, and imaging data. Second, the student must critically examine the initial assessment and *reassess* the patient. In presenting night float patients, Dhaliwal and Hauer recommend that students give "a brief and edited synopsis of the initial data with focus on decision-making, interval reassessments, and systems-based care" [1]. "The provisional diagnosis was _____, but..." is a reasonable way to start the reassessment when the clinical picture looks different in the morning:

> The provisional diagnosis was congestive heart failure, but this morning I'm more concerned about a pulmonary embolism. The onset of dyspnea was acute, there was no weight gain, and the leg edema is asymmetric. The chest x-ray is clear this morning, with no signs of congestion, but the patient continues to be hypoxemic. Also, when we asked him about recent travel this morning, the patient mentioned that he had just returned from London 5 days ago on a transatlantic flight. We've already ordered a stat dose of enoxaparin, and a CT PE protocol.

This case illustrates the importance of reviewing the critical elements of the history with the patient and repeating the key parts of the physical exam. Even if the diagnosis is not in question, a fresh look at the patient and a careful review of overnight events can be extremely helpful. If the student can collect and report the interval data, and start to think critically about the initial assessment, the night float patient can become a teaching and learning opportunity for the whole team.

Transfer Admissions

Transfer admissions are common in teaching hospitals, and medical students can serve a number of useful functions with these challenging patients. First and foremost, data collection is critical. Transfers may arrive with very little in the way of medical records, and the student who can track down, review, and organize the facts of the case into a succinct presentation for morning rounds will be recognized as an important contributor. Making late night phone calls to outside medical record departments, faxing consent forms, and paging through reams of daily progress notes and test results are the diligent student's tasks. In the oral presentation, the timeline of the patient's course at the outside hospital should be the final part of the history of present illness (HPI), concluding with the reason for the transfer:

> She was admitted to Suburban Hospital 12 days ago with acute decompensated heart failure. Her course was complicated by hypotension and acute kidney injury thought to be secondary to cardiorenal syndrome. On hospital days 5, 6, and 8 she received hemodialysis via a femoral catheter. On day 10, she spiked a fever to 102 degrees and was diagnosed with a hospital-acquired pneumonia, for which she was started on vancomycin and piperacillin-tazobactam pending sputum and blood culture results. Over the past 2 days, her urine output has improved to about 60 cc/hr on a furosemide drip, and her creatinine has been downtrending. Her fever has resolved and her respiratory status has been stable. She was transferred to our hospital yesterday at the request of her husband, who wanted her to be closer to home.

The assessment should include a brief (one to two lines) summary of the outside hospital course, a respectful appraisal of the diagnostic work-up and treatment the patient received at the outside hospital, an inventory of any pending or missing clinical data, and a statement of "what needs to be done now for the patient." If the diagnosis is in doubt or the treatment plan seems questionable, this is the time to discuss it and reassess the case:

> We agree with the treatment plan as proposed at Suburban and need to follow up on results of the echocardiogram that was done there on the day of transfer, and the blood and sputum cultures. We will need to optimize her heart failure medicines and transition to an oral antibiotic for the hospital-acquired pneumonia, provided that the blood cultures are negative. Also, she is deconditioned and will probably need short-term rehab in a skilled nursing facility.

Note that transfer admissions may present opportunities for practicing high-value care, especially in the area of redundant testing. "Hospital myopia" is a term for the wasteful practice of repeating tests in one's own hospital that have already been done in another. "Let's get all of our data in one place" or "we're too busy to track down all those test results" are some of the rationalizations that lead to hospital myopia. This kind of thinking is unacceptable in a country where unnecessary medical spending amounts to as much as $750 billion per year [2].

Bedside Presentations

Some attendings prefer to have all of their new admissions presented at the bedside. The rationale for the bedside presentation is to humanize the experience for the medical team and to give full transparency to the patient. In this setting, the patient can become an active participant in the presentation, interjecting comments and questions and describing their symptoms in more detail. The overall structure of the oral presentation is unchanged (see Chap. 2), but the student must remember to avoid medical jargon, try to involve the patient in the discussion, and even let the patient tell parts of the story.

Patients like bedside presentations. In one study, 85% of patients preferred having the oral presentation done at the bedside, even though some did not fully understand the discussion. On the other hand, 95% of students and residents felt more comfortable having such discussions away from the patient [3]. However, students and residents very much like bedside *teaching*, especially for core clinical skills such as history taking, physical examination, and professionalism [4]. In practice, the oral presentation and case discussion usually occur in the hallway or conference room, after which the team goes briefly to the bedside, where the attending talks to the patient and does some teaching. My bedside attending routine includes going over key points in the history ("would you describe again what your chest pain was like?") and physical exam ("let's see if I can hear that soft heart murmur the medical student mentioned to you"). This approach allows the patient to verify the story, ask questions, and discuss their care or whatever else is on their mind. It provides many of the benefits of the bedside presentation without undue stress on the student, for whom presenting a case is difficult enough without worrying about translating medicalese into English for the patient.

The Daily Soap Presentation on Rounds

The daily SOAP presentation on morning rounds is a key performance measure for medical students. A good SOAP presentation is concise, well-organized, and up-to-the-minute in terms of symptoms, physical findings, and test results. It should take less than 2 minutes, even for a complex patient. Pre-rounding is essential: a good rule of thumb is to allow 20 minutes per patient, which is time enough to greet the patient, ask about their symptoms, do a focused physical exam, and check vital signs, I's and O's, and the latest lab and imaging results. The presentation should hold strictly to the SOAP format:

- *Subjective*: How is the patient feeling now? How did they do overnight? Are there any new symptoms, or changes in old symptoms, that are pertinent to the case?
- *Objective*: Always give the latest vital signs (if the morning vitals haven't been recorded when you pre-round, check them yourself!). Identify overnight trends, such as fevers spikes or significant changes in blood pressure, heart rate, respiratory rate, or oxygenation. From the nursing notes, check the weight, calculate the I's and O's for the past 24 h, and check the latest clinimetric data such as CIWA or APACHE scores. Perform a focused physical exam, check for the latest lab and imaging results, and see if consultants have made any new recommendations since yesterday.
- *Assessment and Plan*: Assess the response to treatment. Confirm or reassess the working diagnosis. Discuss any new problems or complications. Finally, propose a *specific* treatment plan for the next 24 h.

Consider the following examples of concise SOAP presentations. Note that there is generally no need to rehash the history or summarize the treatment to date. These are work-ing presentations for work rounds:

> Mr. Wade is feeling better this morning. He was able to lie flat all night and slept well. His leg edema is improved, and he was able to walk to the bathroom without dyspnea. His vital signs are 98.4, 74, 16, 138/70, O2 saturation 93% on room air. His weight is down 8 pounds since admission; I's and O's are negative 1500 cc for the past 24 hours. His JVP is down to 7 cm, lungs are clear, heart regu-lar with no murmur or gallop, and there is trace pretibial and ankle edema. Labs are significant for BUN 21, creatinine 1.3, potassium 3.9, and magnesium 2.4. I think that his heart failure is significantly improved. We can transition him from IV to PO furosemide today, and increase his lisinopril from 10 to 20 mg daily. If he continues to do well we might be able to send him home soon, possibly tomorrow.
>
> Ms. Park spiked a fever to 101.7 overnight, with heavy sweats, nausea, and one episode of vomiting. Her right leg pain was 8/10, and she required two doses of oxycodone overnight to control it. This morning, she is lightheaded and feels a little confused. Vitals are 99.6, 110, 20, 94/56, with O2 saturation 91% on 2 liters. Her lungs are clear, heart regular, abdomen soft and non-tender. The right lower leg is still warm and erythematous, and the erythema has spread proximally almost to the knee, well beyond the ink line from yesterday. She is oriented to place and person but not time, and has difficulty concentrating on questions. Her white count this morning is up to 18,000. I'm concerned that her cellulitis is worsening rapidly, she's delirious, and she might be developing sepsis. I think that we should draw blood cultures, give her a 1-liter IV fluid bolus, and add vancomycin to her antibiotic regimen to cover for MRSA. If the hypotension and confusion do not improve over the next 1-2 hours, we should consider transferring her to the ICU for closer monitoring.

Skills required to deliver a useful and concise SOAP pre-sentation on rounds include accurate data collection, data synthesis, clinical judgment, and knowledge of basic clinical management. These daily presentations can be a great way for teachers to assess their students' progress as they advance from data collectors to synthesizers to logical and decisive clinical thinkers. Good SOAP presentations are also impor-tant for efficient and timely patient care. Students who mas-ter the SOAP presentation on rounds can be a terrific asset to their teams.

Calling a Consultant

The ability to call a consultant is a mark of maturity for a medical student. The call can be intimidating, and students worry that the consultant will be impatient, annoyed, or even hostile as they stumble for the right words. In practice, this is seldom the case. Consultants are generally happy to see patients on the teaching service and gracious about educating the team and pointing out the interesting features of the case. They do expect the caller to have the pertinent clinical information and a clear idea of what is needed from the consultant:

> We have a 26-year-old man who got into a pull-up contest with his buddies, and went overboard. He presented with both arms markedly swollen from wrists to shoulders, with inability to bend his elbows. The arm muscles are exquisitely tender; radial and ulnar pulses are weak but palpable in both wrists. Sensation is normal in the hands. The CPK is 80,000. We've started aggressive IV hydration. We'd like you to see him to rule out compartment syndrome.

This was an actual case at our VA hospital when I was attending a few years ago. The orthopedic resident came in quickly and confirmed that he did not have compartment syndrome. We hydrated him aggressively for several days, and the rhabdomyolysis gradually resolved without any permanent kidney damage. Note that the call sums up the key points of the case in a few sentences and ends with a specific request. Here is another example of a concise presentation for a surgical consultant:

> Mr. Stokes is a 49-year-old man who came to us last night with fever, right upper quadrant pain, and leukocytosis. Ultrasound showed no gallbladder wall-thickening or gallstones; there was some questionable fat stranding. We think he might have acalculous cholecystitis, and we've ordered a HIDA scan. Would you take a look at him, please?

And here is a very specific request for a rheumatologist:

> Ms. Bellflower is a 62-year-old woman with type 2 diabetes who presented with acute monarthritis of the right wrist. On exam, the

wrist is markedly swollen, erythematous, and exquisitely tender. She has a low-grade fever and her WBC is 12,000. We'd like you to tap her wrist to rule out infection and check for crystals.

Consultants do expect certain courtesies. Adherence to the following simple rules can help to minimize friction, enhance education, and maintain a pleasant and enjoyable work environment:

1. Call consults as early in the day as possible.
2. Have pertinent clinical information available; anticipate what will be needed.
3. Be judicious with consults. Nonurgent problems can be dealt with at outpatient visits.
4. Use each consult as a learning opportunity [5].

The Emergency Room Presentation

Even students who have mastered the oral presentation in other settings may struggle when they first work in the emergency room. The atmosphere can be chaotic, with sick patients arriving in bunches and busy, distracted attendings. In this setting, a concise and focused presentation containing all pertinent information is essential. The basic structure of the ER presentation is similar to the oral presentation on the wards, but the mindset is different. As described by Peter Rosen in 1979, it is "the biology of emergency medicine" that demands a different kind of assessment, defined not by organ systems or specific diseases but by "the level of life threat" [6]. The ER presentation should assess for life- or limb-threatening conditions and prioritize the patient's care according to the level of concern. Table 3.1 describes the essential features of the ER oral presentation [7]. I would add that a concise, accurate timeline and rich descriptions of the key symptoms and physical findings are just as important in the ER as on the wards:

The patient is a 47-year-old man with type 2 diabetes, hypertension, and hyperlipidemia with a chief complaint of chest pain off and on for 3 days. On further questioning, he first had the pain

TABLE 3.1 Distinctive features of the emergency room (ER) oral case presentation

Important emergency medicine traits	Recommendations for oral presentations in the ER
Assume every patient has a life-/limb-threatening condition	Be concise. The listener expects the presenter to use clinical judgment to edit patient information, with an emphasis on characteristics that apply to the inclusion or exclusion of life threats
Juggle multiple patients simultaneously	Present in less than 5 min. State CC first and focus only on CC unless other concerning problems arise
Prioritize patients	Only talk about the most pressing issues; as there are multiple patients with pressing issues, focusing a presentation allows for rapid assessment of the critical nature of their complaint and subsequent triage among other patients
Address patient loyalty issues and consequences of incomplete medical records	Obtain a complete history. As patients are not tied to a specific practitioner, "hospital hopping" is more common, meaning a complete picture cannot rely on medical records. Therefore, it is critical to get a detailed interview

Adapted from Davenport et al. [7]. With permission from John Wiley & Sons
CC chief complaint

about 6 weeks ago, when he was loading a truck at work, then had two or three more episodes of exertional pain over the next month. Three days ago, the pain awoke him and has continued to occur every few hours, both with exertion and at rest. The pain is dull, squeezing and substernal with radiation to the left shoulder. It lasts 5-10 minutes and goes away on its own when he rests. He does have diaphoresis and nausea with the pain, but no shortness of breath. The pain is not pleuritic. He tried antacids without relief; he also tried one of his father's nitroglycerin tablets once, and got rapid relief. His meds are aspirin, atorvastatin, metformin, and losartan; he takes them every day. He is a one-pack-per-day smoker; he does not use cocaine or other illicit drugs. He has no prior history of chest pain or cardiac testing. His father had an MI at age 57. On exam, the vital signs are 144/72, 88, 16, 98.7 degrees. O2 saturation is 97% on room air. The jugular venous pressure is 5 cm, and there are no carotid bruits; lungs are clear; heart regular S4S1S2 with no murmurs or rubs; the abdomen is soft and non-tender; there is no leg edema. The metabolic panel is normal, and the troponin is 0.0. ECG reveals sinus rhythm with a right bundle branch block (also seen 2 years ago), and no ST-T abnormalities. His chest x-ray is normal.

To sum up, this is a 47-year-old man with multiple cardiac risk factors and an accelerating pattern of chest pain that is concerning for angina. He's not having chest pain now, but his TIMI score is 3, which means he has a 13% risk of a fatal or nonfatal cardiac event in the next 14 days. We would like to admit him to cardiology for possible heart catheterization tomorrow.

Note that clinimetric risk scales such as TIMI for unstable angina, the Wells score for DVT, and the Ranson criteria for acute pancreatitis can aid in triage and treatment decisions in the ER. Medical students should not hesitate to use these and other validated risk scales in their oral presentations.

The social history is critical in the assessment of emergency room patients. It is important to know, for instance, that a man who needs daily dressing changes for a large perirectal abscess is homeless and has no one to help him with dressing changes and no address to give to the visiting nurse. He might need an advocate to push for him to be hospitalized for his dressing changes. The ER is an important setting for advocacy, because triage decisions are made quickly, and important social factors can be missed by busy physicians who are juggling many patients. Medical students should recognize that they can (and must) become advocates for their patients.

The Outpatient Clinic Presentation

In the outpatient clinic, students must learn to present new patients, routine follow-ups, and patients coming in with urgent problems. This requires a versatile approach to the oral presentation. New patients generally require a complete history and physical, which (like the admission H&P for hospitalized patients) serves as a complete archive of the patient's baseline health status at the time of the visit. Follow-up patient presentations should include a brief interval history, an update on the status of the major conditions on their problem list (with pertinent positives and negatives), a focused physical exam, and a concise, problem-based assessment and plan. For example, the presentation of a patient with hypertension, type 2 diabetes mellitus and congestive heart failure might go as follows:

Mr. Hough is a 69-year-old man with hypertension, type 2 DM, and CHF, here today for routine follow-up. He hasn't had any hospitalizations or ER visits over the past 3 months. His main complaint today is moderate fatigue, which he describes as a low energy level, not excessive sleepiness. He does not have constipation, myalgias, orthostatic symptoms, or cold intolerance. He is mostly sedentary, and does very little walking or other exercise. His weight is stable since his last visit; he sleeps on one pillow and is not having PND. He gets mild ankle edema as the day goes on, which is typically better by the next morning. He is not having any chest pain or palpitations; he's short of breath walking a half block or climbing one flight of stairs, as before. He takes metformin and glipizide for his diabetes, and his fasting glucoses have ranged from 85-160 recently; pre-supper glucoses are higher, generally 160-200. He had mild hypoglycemic symptoms once last week when he was late for lunch, and took a couple of glucose tablets with rapid relief. He also complains of a painful callus on the bottom of his left foot. His home blood pressures have ranged from 130-150/80-90 recently; he takes all of his medicines every day. The rest of the review of systems was unremarkable. Today, his blood pressure was 152/94 initially, and 138/88 when I repeated it after 10 minutes at rest. O2 saturation is 97% on room air. His JVP is normal at 6 cm, and there is no cervical lymphadenopathy or thyromegaly; the lungs are clear, and the heart is regular with an S4 gallop but no murmurs. The abdomen is soft and nontender, with no masses or organomegaly. There is trace pretibial edema bilaterally. On foot exam, there is a 2x2 cm plantar callus beneath the first MTP joint on the left foot, with no surrounding erythema, warmth, fluctuance, or discharge. The DP and PT pulses are 1+ bilaterally. Monofilament sensation is absent in both feet. Labs are significant for a hemoglobin A1c of 7.8% 4 months ago, with normal CBC, renal function and electrolytes but an elevated urine microalbum/creatinine ratio of 87.4 at that time. His last TSH was 4.5 2 years ago.

Assessment and Plan:

#1. HTN is not adequately controlled. His target BP level is <130/80. Since he has microalbuminuria and is on only 10 mg lisinopril daily, I think we should increase the lisinopril to 20 mg daily and schedule a nurse BP check in 2-3 weeks.

#2. CHF is compensated, NYHA functional class II, and the patient appears euvolemic on exam.

#3. Type 2 diabetes mellitus, ? control. With his longstanding diabetes, his target HA1c is around 7.5%. Some of his recent fasting and pre-supper glucoses are above the target range. We need to recheck his hemoglobin A1c today, and consider adjusting his medications if it is >7.5%.

#4. Plantar callus, left foot. There are no signs of infection, but with his lack of sensation he is at high risk for developing a foot ulcer. He needs to see podiatry within a week to treat the callus.

#5. Fatigue, cause unclear. Possibly due to deconditioning, but will check TSH (which was high-normal 2 years ago), renal panel, AM cortisol, and CBC. Plan to start him on a gentle aerobic exercise program and gradually increase his activity.

#6. Health maintenance. He is up to date on all immunizations. He had a single tubular adenoma on his screening colonoscopy 2 years ago, and is due for follow-up in 3 years. He has a 30-pack-year smoking history and quit 10 years ago; he is not interested in lung cancer screening.

Plan:

Lab testing as above. Increase lisinopril to 20 mg daily. Podiatry referral. Nurse BP check in 2-3 weeks. See me in 3 months.

Note that an accurate and updated problem list is essential for both oral presentations and progress notes on follow-up patients. A common mistake is to include *every* problem on the list in the oral presentation, including the inactive and irrelevant ones. This leads to an overly long presentation with too much information for the attending to process. The same goes for progress notes, where endless problem lists are cut and pasted into the assessment (this practice almost makes me long for the old days of the paper chart – at least those written assessments were concise!). When you present your follow-up patient, *edit the problem list to include only the active and relevant issues for that visit.* The above patient might have gout, chronic low back pain, and a history of achalasia, but if they are not active issues, they should not be part of the oral presentation.

The presentation of a patient with an urgent complaint should center on the reason for the visit, with a concise HPI that includes a timeline of the complaint, a limited physical exam, and a brief assessment and plan:

> The patient is a 28-year-old man with no chronic medical problems who presents with a tender "knot" on his abdomen for 3 days. He thinks it is getting larger, and it is tender to the touch. He does not recall any insect bites, or other trauma to the area. He does not have fevers or chills. On exam, he's afebrile with normal vital signs. There is a 2x2 cm firm, movable lump in the left lower abdomen that is tender, red, and slightly warm, with no fluctuance or discharge. I think it's a furuncle. Since there's no evidence of an abscess at this point, I'd like to treat him with warm compresses and a 5-day course of trimethoprim-sulfamethoxazole to cover for methicillin-resistant Staph aureus. If it comes to a head and an abscess develops, he'll need to come in to the ER for an I&D.

Note the laser-like focus for the urgent presentation, although this would change if his blood pressure were 190/120 or if he complained of chest pain on the way out the door.

The SNAPPS Presentation

The outpatient clinic is often a passive learning setting for medical students. Clinic preceptors are busy, with too many patients to see and too little time for teaching. When a student presents a case, the preceptor will usually make a couple of teaching points and then dictate a treatment plan, with very little discussion. SNAPPS [8], a "learner-centered model for medical education," was devised to encourage medical students to take an active role in the office or outpatient clinic and express their thinking and reasoning (Table 3.2). SNAPPS stresses the importance of asking questions and engaging preceptors with an interactive case discussion. The preceptor, of course, must learn and understand the SNAPPS approach and accept the challenges and pleasures of the Socratic dialogues that it engenders. For preceptors, another nice thing about SNAPPS is that it relieves them of the pressure to think up new teaching points. For students, there is nothing better than active case-based learning. Consider a

TABLE 3.2 SNAPPS: a learner-centered model for outpatient education

S	Summarize briefly the history and findings
N	Narrow the differential to two or three relevant possibilities
A	Analyze the differential, comparing and contrasting the possibilities
P	Probe the preceptor by asking questions about uncertainties, difficulties, or alternative approaches
P	Plan management for the patient's medical issues
S	Select a case-related issue for self-directed learning

Reprinted with permission from Wolpaw et al. [8], https://journals.lww.com/academicmedicine/pages/default.aspx

SNAPPS-style discussion of Mr. Hough's complaint of fatigue in the above scenario:

Student: I was thinking about the differential diagnosis for his fatigue. He could have hypothyroidism. His TSH was high-normal 2 years ago, and he's very tired, but he doesn't have weight gain, constipation, or cold intolerance. I wonder if those symptoms are always present with hypothyroidism?

Preceptor: I don't know about always, but my impression is that patients with the classic symptoms in addition to fatigue are much more likely to have hypothyroidism.

Student: Interesting…that might be a good thing for me to look up. Against adrenal insufficiency, he's not lightheaded when he stands up, and there is no hyperpigmentation.

Preceptor: So adrenal insufficiency is probably less likely. What else are you thinking about?

Student: Well, he might have anemia. He hasn't had any melena or hematochezia, but he did have one tubular adenoma removed when he had his colonoscopy 2 years ago. He doesn't seem to have pallor. His hemoglobin was normal 6 months ago.

Preceptor:	How about other types of anemia?
Student:	Do you mean anemia of chronic disease? Associated with malignancy or infection? He doesn't have any obvious symptoms...
Preceptor:	Does he have shoulder and hip pain and stiffness as well as fatigue?
Student:	Oh, you're thinking of....
Preceptor:	Polymyalgia rheumatica.
Student:	Well, he didn't complain of that; I'd like to go back and ask him about it. But all in all, I think the most likely thing is deconditioning. He's been very inactive for a long time. He gets tired with modest physical activity, but his heart failure seems to be well-compensated. I think he might benefit from an aerobic exercise program through cardiac rehab.
Preceptor:	That sounds good, but I would go ahead with the lab work-up you suggested – the TSH, CBC, electrolytes, AM cortisol, and an ESR if he does turn out to have shoulder and hip girdle pain and stiffness.
Student:	OK, and I'll read more about hypothyroidism in the absence of classic symptoms, and let you know what I find tomorrow [9].
Preceptor:	Let's go see him together.

References

1. Dhaliwal G, Hauer KE. The oral patient presentation in the era of night float admissions. Credit and critique. JAMA. 2013;310(21):2247–8.
2. Institute of Medicine. The healthcare imperative: lowering costs and improving outcomes. Washington, DC: The National Academies Press; 2010.
3. Wang-Cheng R, Barnas GP, Sigmann P, Riendl PA, Young MJ. Bedside case presentations. Why patients like them but learners don't. J Gen Intern Med. 1989;4:284–7.
4. Gonzalo JD, Masters PA, Simons RJ, Chuang CH. Attending rounds and bedside case presentations: medical student and

medicine resident experiences and attitudes. Teach Learn Med. 2009;21(2):105–10.

5. Bly RA, Bly EG. Consult courtesy. J Grad Med Educ. 2013;5(3):533–4.

6. Rosen P. The biology of emergency medicine. J Am Coll Emerg Phys. 1979;8:280–3.

7. Davenport C, Honigman B, Druck J. The 3-minute emergency medicine medical student presentation: a variation on a theme. Acad Emerg Med. 2008;15(7):683–7.

8. Wolpaw TM, Wolpaw DR, Papp KK. SNAPPS: a learner-centered model for outpatient education. Acad Med. 2003;78(9):893–8.

9. Canaris GJ, Steiner JF, Ridgway EC. Do traditional symptoms of hypothyroidism correlate with biochemical disease? J Gen Intern Med. 1997;12(9):544–50.

Chapter 4
The HPI: A Timeline, Not a Time Machine

Chronology…is crucial. The time machine delivery, where the speaker begins now, traces backwards, and skips ahead, leaves listeners lost in space.

Kurt Kroenke

In the HPI, try not to flip back and forth between pain and diarrhea.

Attending feedback to a third-year medical student

The Timeline, from Hippocrates to Lawrence Weed

There is nothing new about our use of a timeline in the history of present illness (HPI). In his *Epidemics* (c. 400 BC), Hippocrates made meticulous use of timelines in his day-by-day descriptions of disease:

A woman, who lodged on the Quay, being three months gone with child, was seized with fever, and immediately began to have pains in the loins. On the third day, pain of the head and neck, extending to the clavicle, and right hand; she immediately lost the power of speech; was paralyzed in the right hand, with spasms, after the manner of paraplegia; was quite incoherent; passed an uncomfortable night; did not sleep; disorder of the bowels, attended with bilious. On the fourth, recovered the use of her tongue; spasms of the same parts, and general pains remained; swelling in the hypochondrium, accompanied with pain; did not sleep, was quite incoherent; bowels disordered, urine thin, and not

© Springer Nature Switzerland AG 2019
C. D. Packer, *Presenting Your Case*,
https://doi.org/10.1007/978-3-030-13792-2_4

of a good color. On the fifth, acute fever; pain of the hypochondrium, quite incoherent; alvine evacuations bilious; towards night
had a sweat, and was freed from the fever. On the sixth, recovered
her reason; was every way relieved; the pain remained about the
left clavicle; was thirsty, urine thin, had no sleep. On the seventh
trembling, slight coma, some incoherence, pains about the clavicle
and left arm remained; in all other respects was alleviated; quite
coherent. For 3 days remained free from fever. On the eleventh,
had a relapse, with rigor and fever. About the fourteenth day,
vomited pretty abundantly bilious and yellow matters, had a
sweat, the fever went off, by coming to a crisis. [1]

Hippocrates knew that the complex natural histories of
the diseases he observed could only be reported with careful
and accurate chronologies. In the above case, he describes a
14-day illness with a fluctuating course of fever, headache,
neck and clavicular pain, neurologic symptoms, abdominal
pain, diarrhea, and vomiting. The timeline makes the description comprehensible. This is a common thread as we read the
case histories of Paracelsus, Rhazes, Sydenham, Addison,
Graves, Parkinson, Laennec, Charcot, Virchow, Osler, Reed,
Cushing, etc.; all are marked by careful chronological descriptions of symptoms. Consider Thomas Sydenham's classic
seventeenth-century description of measles:

The measles generally attack children. On the first day they have
chills and shivers, and are hot and cold in turns. On the second
they have the fever in full – disquietude, thirst, want of appetite, a
white (but not dry) tongue, slight cough, heaviness of the head
and eyes, and somnolence. The nose and eyes run continually; and
this is the surest sign of measles...The symptoms increase until
the fourth day. *Then* – or sometimes on the fifth – there appear
on the face and forehead small red spots, very like the bites of
fleas. These increase in number, and cluster together, so as to
mark the face with large red blotches. They are formed by small
papulae, so slightly elevated above the skin, that their prominence
can hardly be detected by the eye, but can just be felt by passing
the fingers lightly along the skin. The spots take hold of the face
first; from which they spread to the chest and belly, and after-
wards to the legs and ankles...On the sixth day, or thereabouts,
the forehead and face begin to grow rough, as the pustules die off,
and as the skin breaks. Over the rest of the body the blotches are
both very broad and very red. About the eighth day they
disappear from the face, and scarcely show on the rest of the body.

On the ninth, there are none anywhere. On the face, however, and on the extremities – sometimes over the trunk – they peel off in thin, mealy squamulae; at which time the fever, the difficulty of breathing, and the cough are aggravated. [2]

It is precisely this kind of rich chronological description that that modern medical students need to incorporate into their oral presentations. This notion, again, is nothing new; according to the "Form of Medical History and Physical Examination" of the University Hospitals of Cleveland Department of Medicine (1945), students recording the present illness should:

...try to give a concise, logical story of the development of the patient's illness with dates of the onset of important symptoms. Do not record events in the order in which the patient tells them, but in order of their occurrence. Discuss the character of onset and the earliest symptoms noticed; describe the series of events leading up to his admission to the clinic.

The anonymous author of the handbook continues in a cautionary vein:

A student's first attempts at writing a P.I. often result in a document characterized by a poorly organized list of disorganized symptoms. This sketchy quality is less likely to occur if one thinks of possible diseases which are suggested as the story unfolds. New questions are thereby brought to mind and a more intelligent interrogation of the patient is permitted. [3]

A clear timeline is prerequisite for the kind of "intelligent interrogation" the author suggests. The natural history of any disease is recognizable as a series of events, and if the order of events is not accurately recorded in the HPI, diagnosis can be difficult.

Dr. Lawrence Weed was a physician and biochemist who became frustrated with the haphazard and careless "ink splashes" and "private scribbles" that passed for medical progress notes in his day [4]. He saw the necessity for a new form of physician record-keeping that would combine the scientific rigor of his basic science research with a more useful and organized version of the medical record. Weed's "problem-oriented medical record," first proposed in a 1964

Irish Journal of Medical Science article, has now become the worldwide standard in both medical care and medical education. In that article, Weed comments on the importance of an accurate chronology of events and data (using tables or graphs if necessary) and the need for a flexible format for the HPI:

> The present illness should be a statement of the relevant facts about a problem or series of problems.... When the story is long and the data voluminous, a table or a graph should be constructed. The graph or table should be so organised that the data collected during the hospital stay or following it, can be added at the time the data are acquired. In chronic disease particularly, the hospital stay should not be treated as an isolated incident, but rather as an opportunity to get, under more controlled conditions, a few more points on already established curves...*Enslavement to the conventional format of the medical history can make a problem almost incomprehensible by separating the pertinent facts, putting some in the past history, some under laboratory data and some in the systems review* [emphasis added]. [4]

Weed's insights apply nicely when we consider the case of a patient with Crohn's disease on the immunosuppressive drug azathioprine (AZA) who was repeatedly admitted for fever, leukocytosis, arthralgias, rash, and LFT abnormalities. Infectious causes were ruled out; the arthralgias and rash raised concern for extraintestinal manifestations of his Crohn's disease, but the symptoms improved spontaneously in each instance without any specific IBD treatment:

> Ultimately, it was only after the third admission with still no evidence of an infectious etiology that the possibility of AZA hypersensitivity was considered in earnest. The association became clear by aligning the timing of his fevers with the timing of AZA ingestion. Further evidence of AZA hypersensitivity included clear clinical improvement each time the AZA was stopped and the escalating clinical and laboratory manifestations that occurred with each rechallenge. This intensifying response with each exposure is a hallmark of hypersensitivity reactions. [5]

In this case, a graph with the timing of the fever spikes in relation to administration of his medicines would have made the temporal relationship clear and might have led to an earlier diagnosis of azathioprine hypersensitivity. In Weed's terminology, the "pertinent facts were presented separately," and the critical relationship was not seen until the third hospitalization.

To illustrate the importance of an integrated HPI, consider the hypothetical case of a man who was admitted with 3 days of nausea, vomiting, and abdominal pain and found to be in ketoacidosis with an anion gap of 30 and a glucose of 250. He was started on an insulin drip and shortly thereafter became severely hypoglycemic. In retrospect, the key fact that had been missing from the timeline was that he had been on a 2-day alcohol bender prior to the onset of symptoms and was a frequent binge drinker. This information had been included in the social history, but was not reported in the HPI. The correct diagnosis in this case was alcoholic ketoacidosis, not diabetic ketoacidosis. Aggressive rehydration with D5 normal saline was the only treatment required. The inappropriate insulin drip could have been avoided with a more integrated history and a complete chronology of events.

Case Reports and the Importance of the Timeline

Case reports can give us many insights into the importance of a well-integrated HPI with a clear and complete timeline. Many case reports use graphs and tables to reveal the chronological details of the clinical course and the interrelatedness of events. Figure 4.1 gives the clinical timeline of a 7-year-old girl with bubonic plague, including key events and symptoms, diagnostic work-up, antibiotic treatment, ICU course, and eventual recovery [6]. Figure 4.2 gives the timeline of a 72-year-old man with gastric cancer who developed unexpected isolated adrenocorticotropic hormone deficiency (IAD) during chemotherapy [7]. At first he was treated presumptively for SIADH with fluid restriction, with no improvement in either his electrolyte abnormalities or his generalized fatigue and anorexia. Once the diagnosis was made, the administration of hydrocortisone dramatically

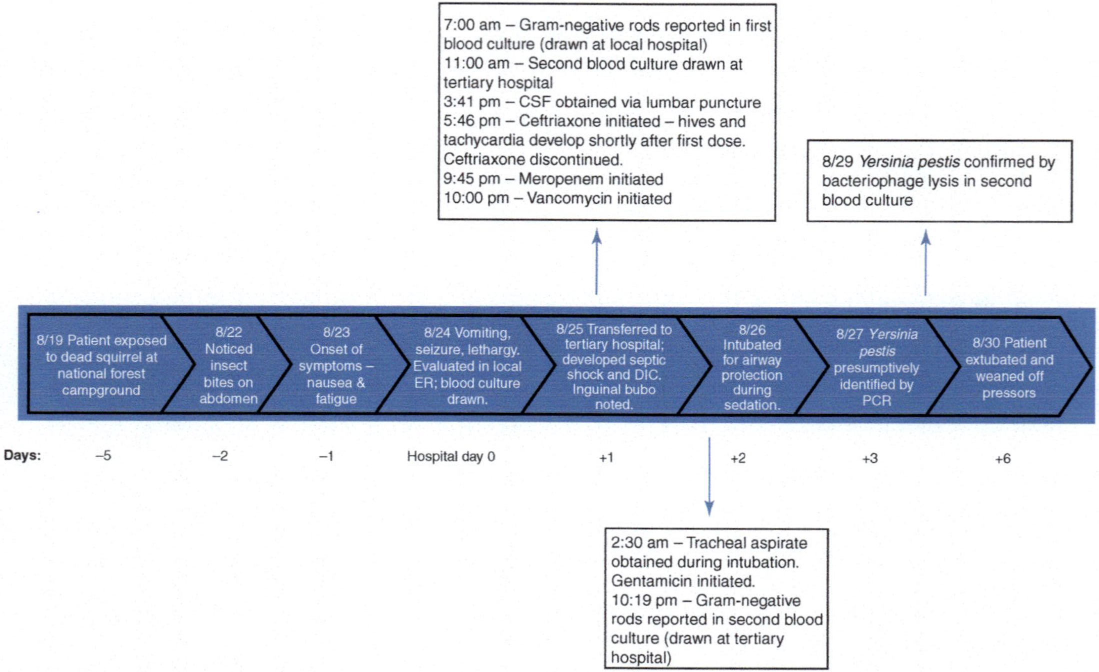

FIGURE 4.1 Timeline of events for a 7-year-old girl with bubonic plague [6]. *CSF* Cerebrospinal fluid, *DIC* disseminated intravascular coagulation. (From Drummond et al. [6], by permission of Oxford University Press)

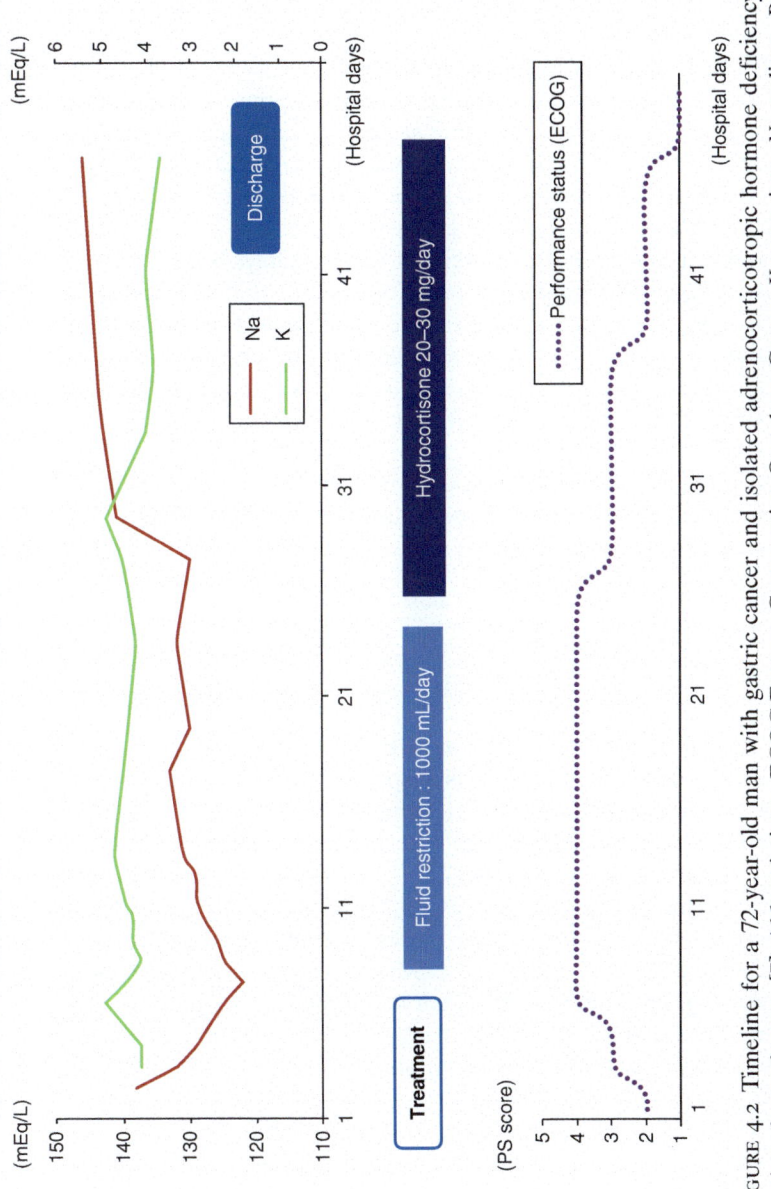

FIGURE 4.2 Timeline for a 72-year-old man with gastric cancer and isolated adrenocorticotropic hormone deficiency during chemotherapy [7]. Abbreviations: *ECOG* Eastern Cooperative Oncology Group, *K* potassium, *Na* sodium, *PS* performance status. (Copyright © Kinoshita et al. [7]; licensee BioMed Central Ltd. 2014)

improved the patient's hyponatremia and boosted his performance status.

In both cases, the clinical timeline shows more than the
natural history of the disease and the response to treatment:
it implicitly reveals the clinical decision-making and clinical
reasoning, and it calls for a hypothesis to explain the events
of the case. In the report of the patient with gastric cancer and
IAD, the authors note that powerful stressors such as external wounds, infection, surgery, or bleeding have been reported
to trigger IAD; they go on to speculate that the stress of
febrile neutropenia might have precipitated IAD in their
patient. Every element of a successful oral presentation – an
accurate timeline, rich and focused descriptions of the key
findings, and an assessment that puts the case in context and
explains what happened – can be found in a high-quality case
report. It follows that medical students who are interesting in
learning to present their patients well should read as many
case reports as possible.

The Timeline as "Origin Story"
for the Chief Complaint

You admit a 73-year-old man with 2 days of nausea, vomiting,
and abdominal pain, who is suspected to have a small bowel
obstruction (SBO). On reviewing his history you realize that
the timeline for his present illness (Fig. 4.3) stretches back to
15 years before admission:

Think of the timeline as an "origin story" for the chief
complaint. The story of this patient's small bowel obstruction
did not begin 2 days before admission, when he developed
nausea and vomiting. It began in 2003 when he underwent a
hemicolectomy for colon cancer, which was the probable
underlying cause of his hospitalization for lysis of adhesions
7 years later, which led in turn to his subsequent episodes of
SBO. The implications of this history are important: a conservative approach is preferred in a patient with multiple
abdominal surgeries and recurrent SBO episodes. More

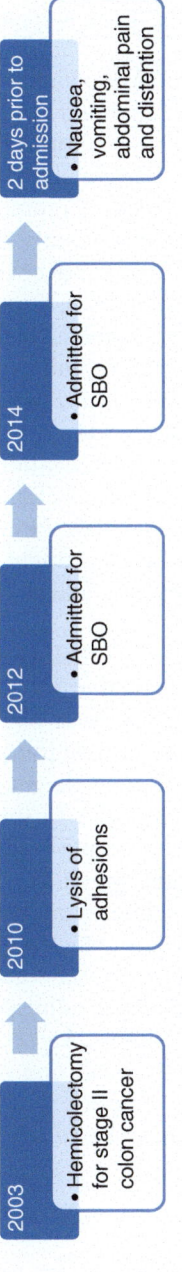

FIGURE 4.3 Clinical timeline for a 73-year-old man with nausea, vomiting, and abdominal pain

surgery would only create more adhesions, and increase the risk for future problems.

Similarly, consider the case of a 48-year-old woman with decompensated alcoholic cirrhosis (MELD score 23) admitted for alcohol detox and intractable ascites. In reviewing the history, you find that the "origin story" for this patient's cirrhosis begins with an episode of military sexual trauma she suffered in her 20s. She subsequently developed PTSD and began to drink heavily, which led over the years to numerous admissions for alcohol withdrawal, seizures, and delirium tremens. More recently, she had an episode of upper GI bleeding and was diagnosed with gastric and esophageal varices. Her clinical timeline (Fig. 4.4) is a harrowing story of the effects of untreated PTSD and severe alcoholism:

In this case, the important implication of the history is that this patient desperately needs treatment for her military sexual trauma and PTSD. It might be too late to reverse the course of her cirrhosis, but treatment of her psychic pain might help her to stop drinking and stabilize her liver disease enough to be considered for transplant.

In some acute illnesses, the timeline may begin days, hours, or even minutes before arrival at the hospital. Consider the case of a previously healthy 66-year-old man (Fig. 4.5), who is admitted with fever and acute respiratory symptoms:

This patient was eventually diagnosed with pneumonia due to *Streptococcus pneumoniae*, a severe illness with mortality as high as 30% when complicated by sepsis. The abrupt onset with high fever, shaking chills, and dense lobar infiltrates is typical of pneumococcal pneumonia, so the timeline in this case gives us important clues as to the etiology.

A good practice for a third-year student is to sketch out a rough clinical timeline for every admission and use it to present the history of present illness. A good timeline will help to keep the oral presentation linear and focused. Furthermore, the "origin story" of the present illness helps the team to see the big picture and understand the context of the illness in the patient's life.

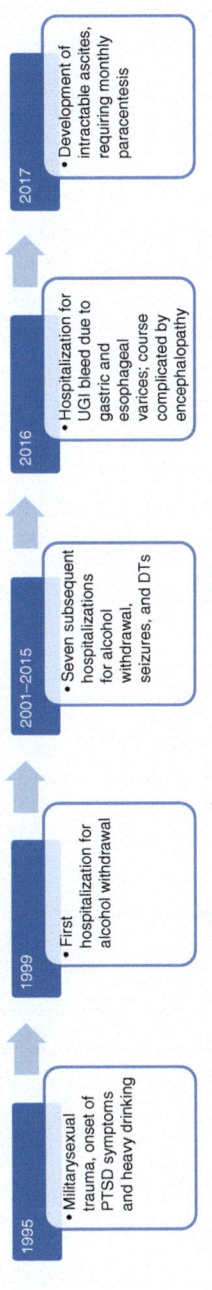

FIGURE 4.4 Clinical timeline for a 48-year-old woman with alcoholic cirrhosis

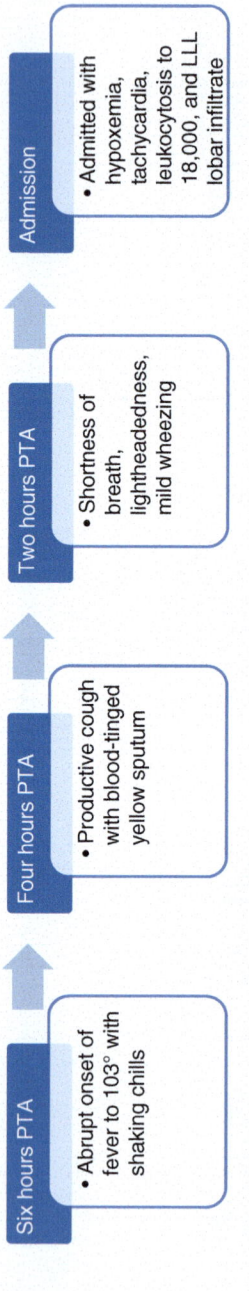

FIGURE 4.5 Clinical timeline for a 66-year-old man with acute respiratory symptoms

The Clinical Flow Sheet

In his landmark 1968 article, "Medical Records that Guide and Teach," Lawrence Weed comments:

> Flow sheets should not be limited to patients with acute problems. Many chronic difficulties are best understood and managed by relation of multiple variables over time – daily, weekly, or monthly. Patients with hypertension, diabetes, and renal and liver disease are among the many who require well structured and up-to-date flow sheets. [8]

Table 4.1 presents clinical data for a 19-year-old American football player who developed intractable muscle cramping immediately after 10 minutes of cold water immersion following a strenuous full-contact football practice. He was diagnosed with rhabdomyolysis and acute kidney injury, which resolved with IV hydration and potassium repletion. This clinical flow sheet gives key laboratory data that show the rapid resolution of the patient's acute kidney injury, and the more gradual downtrending of his creatine kinase and myoglobin levels. The authors of the case report hypothesize that the intense exercise combined with the extreme temperature shift of the cold water bath triggered the muscle trauma and conclude that cold water immersion, thought to speed muscle recovery, might actually increase risk for muscle trauma after heavy exertion.

The clinical flow sheet allows clinicians to see and understand the dynamics of a case, the physiologic forces that underlie the clinical timeline. Table 4.2 is a flow sheet for a patient hospitalized with congestive heart failure. It helps us to comprehend the complex interplay of physiology and pharmacology in this challenging disease.

For the experienced physician, the clinical flow chart reads like the score of a symphony. As we view the data, the harmonics and dissonances of the case play out in our minds. In other words, to push the analogy further, we hear the music of the case. We begin to understand how everything fits together.

TABLE 4.1 Exertional rhabdomyolysis in a collegiate American football player after preventive cold-water immersion [9]

| Date and time | | | | | | |
Biochemical marker	August 9, 2:34 PM	August 9, 6:55 PM	August 9, 11:30 PM	August 10, 5:05 AM	August 14, 1:17 PM	Normal limits[a]
Creatine kinase, IU/L	2545	2352	2661	2668	999	0–190
Myoglobin, ng/mL	499	680	354	190	118	0–149
Potassium, mEq/L	3.2	4.2	4	4.5	4.4	3.3–5.3
Total carbon dioxide content, mEq/L	23	27.7	26.7	29.2	29.8	23.0–29.0
Chloride, mEq/L	95	106	106	108	99	100–112
Glucose, mg/dL	180	83	97	87	98	70–125
Creatinine, mg/dL	1.6	1.2	1.1	1	1.1	0.5–1.4
Calcium, mg/dL	10.7	8.7	9	8.9	10.5	8.5–10.5

Reprinted with permission from Kahanov et al. [9]
[a]Provided by the laboratory for the general population

TABLE 4.2 Medical student flow sheet for a congestive heart failure patient

Date	6/8	6/9	6/10	6/11	6/12	6/13	6/14	6/15
BP	98/60	94/62	105/70	102/66	112/74	116/68	124/70	128/74
Wt (kg)	93.2	91.8	90.4	89.3	88.9	88.0	87.2	87.0
I/O (cc)	−1900	−2000	−1500	−1200	−800	−800	−600	−200
Na	128	127	129	131	133	135	134	134
K	3.1	3.3	3.8	3.6	4.1	4.4	3.5	3.8
Creatinine	1.6	1.7	1.5	1.3	1.2	1.2	1.3	1.1
JVP (cm)	14	12	10	10	9	8	8	6
Rales	½ up	½ up	¼ up	¼ up	Bibasilar	Bibasilar	–	–
LE edema	3+	2+	2+	2+	1+	1+	Trace	Trace
O$_2$ sat %	88–90	93	91	93	92	90	91	94
FiO$_2$	0.50	0.50	0.32	0.32	0.28	0.24	0.21	0.21
Furosemide dose (mg)	80 IV bid	40 IV bid	40 IV bid	40 IV	40 IV	40 PO bid	40 PO bid	40 PO
Lisinopril dose (mg)	5	5	10	10	20	20	20	20

The electronic health record now enables us to construct elaborate flow sheets with a few mouse clicks, and there is no longer any excuse for missing the trends and interrelated events that used to elude us. Medical students should create and maintain clinical flow sheets for their patients, adding on new data points daily. In addition to guiding clinical decision-making, these flow sheets can help tremendously with the student's daily SOAP presentation on rounds (see Chap. 3) and stimulate useful case discussions. Thinking about the flow sheet data leads naturally to theorizing about cause and effect, reassessing the trajectory of the case, and modifying treatment plans.

Seven Keys to Presenting the HPI

1. Sketch out a timeline for every patient you admit, and use it when you present the HPI.
2. Keep the timeline linear; start at the beginning, and move forward. It's a timeline, not a time machine.
3. Learn the "origin story" for the chief complaint, the true onset of the problem, and start the history from there.
4. Tell the story well: give rich and detailed descriptions of the key events and symptoms over time.
5. Liberate yourself from enslavement to the conventional form of the medical history. All pertinent facts should be presented together in the HPI. When the facts are presented separately, the problem becomes almost incomprehensible.
6. Create a flow sheet for your patients with complex illnesses and multiple data points that need to be followed over time. Update the flow sheet daily, and refer to it when you present your patients on rounds.
7. Try to present the HPI from memory. Telling a story is more effective – and almost always more fluent and concise – than reading from notes.

References

1. The Internet Classics Archive. Hippocrates: of the epidemics (trans: Adams F). 1994. http://classics.mit.edu/Hippocrates/epidemics.1.i.html. Accessed 10 June 2018.
2. Latham RG (trans.). The works of Thomas Sydenham. Volume II, London: Sydenham Society; 1850.
3. Anonymous. Form of medical history and physical examination. University Hospitals of Cleveland Department of Medicine; 1945. p. 1–2.
4. Weed LL. Medical records, patient care, and medical education. Ir J Med Sci. 1964;462:271–82.
5. Mookherjee S, Narayanan M, Uchiyama T, Wentworth KL. Three hospital admissions in 9 days to diagnose azathioprine hypersensitivity in a patient with Crohn's disease. Am J Ther. 2015;22(2):e28–32.
6. Drummond WK, Nelson CA, Fowler J, Epson EE, Mead PS, Lawaczeck EW. Plague in a pediatric patient: case report and use of polymerase chain reaction as a diagnostic aid. J Pediatr Infect Dis Soc. 2014;3(4):e38–41.
7. Kinoshita J, Higashino S, Fushida S, Oyama K, Watanabe T, Okamoto K, et al. Isolated adrenocorticotropic hormone deficiency development during chemotherapy for gastric cancer: a case report. J Med Case Rep. 2014;8:90.
8. Weed LL. Medical records that guide and teach. N Engl J Med. 1968;278(11):593–600.
9. Kahanov L, Eberman LE, Wasik M, Alvey T. Exertional rhabdomyolysis in a collegiate American football player after preventive cold-water immersion: a case report. J Athl Train. 2012;47(2):228–32.

Chapter 5
Pertinent Positives and Negatives

The Role of Pertinent Positives and Negatives in the Oral Presentation

The oral presentation begins with the chief complaint and then a timeline that describes the course of the illness and the interrelatedness of events. Next come the pertinent positives and negatives. The pertinent positives help to make the argument for a particular diagnosis, using the classic signs and symptoms of the disease. The more of these classic findings are present, the more likely the diagnosis. The pertinent negatives help to rule out alternatives to the leading diagnosis while also showing that a thorough differential diagnosis has been considered. Pertinent positives are generally learned by rote, with experience and repetition. Pertinent negatives include both the expected positives that are *not* present (e.g., a patient with signs of decompensated heart failure but no weight gain) and findings that, *by their absence*, help to rule out alternative diagnoses (e.g., a patient with fever and productive cough, with *no dysuria, abdominal pain, or neck stiffness*). Pertinent negatives are not learned by rote; they are derived from the differential diagnosis, which requires a higher order of analytical and creative thinking. Together, the pertinent positives and negatives, like the adjustment knobs of a microscope, bring the diagnosis into focus.

The important thing for the novice presenter to realize is that the argument for a diagnosis begins with the history of present illness (HPI) and that pertinent data must be culled from all of the historical data, including the past medical and surgical history, medications, allergies, family history, social history, and review of systems, and then presented in logical sequence in the HPI. This sounds simple, but selecting the truly pertinent positives and negatives (and leaving out the red herrings) requires careful thought, experience, and clinical judgment. It is also important to understand that the argument for the diagnosis and the ranking of the differential are *implicit* in the HPI, based on how the data are edited, organized, and presented. The *explicit* argument occurs later, in the assessment, with phrases such as "The most likely diagnosis is…" and "The differential diagnosis includes…" In other words, the HPI is more than the story of an illness: using the timeline and the pertinent positives and negatives, it builds the diagnostic framework for the assessment.

Learning the Pertinent Positives

Pertinent positives are learned, memorized, and internalized in the normal process of medical education. With experience and repetition, the pertinent positives for many symptoms and diseases are securely stored in the memory and can be recalled without effort. Asthma, for instance, is associated with wheezing, dyspnea, reversibility, response to bronchodilators, and triggers such as cold air, exercise, allergens, and respiratory infections. Kidney stones cause colicky back, flank, or groin pain, hematuria, dysuria, nausea, and vomiting; 80% are radiopaque, and stones >5 mm in size are unlikely to pass spontaneously. Osteoarthritis of the hip causes groin pain that radiates to the anterior thigh, worsens with weight bearing, and is relieved with rest. Pericarditis presents with sharp, stabbing chest pain that is worse with deep breathing and lying flat, and better with sitting up and leaning forward; electrocardiogram findings include diffuse ST elevation and

PR depression. Celiac disease is associated with chronic diarrhea, weight loss, gluten intolerance, dermatitis herpetiformis, iron deficiency anemia, and tissue transglutaminase antibodies. As an internist with 30 years' experience, I can rattle off these pertinent positives with no effort at all. As a new third-year medical student, you would be well advised to create lists of the pertinent positives for all of the diagnoses you encounter and refer to them often. Remember that Hippocrates taught medicine with aphorisms – pithy observations that contain a general truth – because they are a useful and memorable way to convey medical knowledge. Pertinent positives are the aphorisms of modern medicine. "Chest pain that is substernal, exertional, and relieved with nitroglycerin is angina pectoris" is a great way to remember the three key pertinent positives for anginal chest pain. For medical students, the threefold experience of seeing a patient, reading about the findings, and presenting the patient on rounds works wonders in committing the pertinent positives to memory.

Cases with Pertinent Positives and Negatives

In the following case of a 53-year-old man with chest pain, pertinent positives for the presumed diagnosis of angina pectoris are given in bold print.

Case 1: Chest Pain

A **53-year-old man** with **hypertension, type 2 DM**, and **hyperlipidemia** presents with 3 months of **exertional chest pain**. At first, it occurred only with heavy exertion, such as walking rapidly up a hill or climbing three flights of stairs, but for the past 2 weeks, it has been happening when he **walks 50 ft** or climbs a **half flight of stairs**. The chest pain is **substernal, radiates to the neck and left arm**, and is associated with **nausea, diaphoresis**, and **shortness of breath**. He has not tried sublingual nitroglycerin for the pain. He never had chest pain before 3 months ago and has had no past cardiac testing.

- Medications: He recently had his losartan dose reduced because of low blood pressure. He takes aspirin 81 mg daily but has never been prescribed a statin. He takes OTC saw palmetto for BPH symptoms.
- Family history: His **father had an MI at age 49** and **died of colon cancer at age 63**. His mother has HTN and died of a CVA at age 77. His sister was treated for leukemia at age 32.
- Social history: He is a **one pack per day smoker for 35 years**; he drinks two to three beers per day. He last used cocaine 20 years ago. He smokes marijuana occasionally. He works as a machinist.
- Review of systems:

  – Chronic low back pain, worse lately; occasional right knee pain and swelling.
  – Allergic rhinitis, takes OTC loratadine.
  – **Intermittent black stool for the past 3 months**.
  – Slow stream, nocturia × 3 lately.
  – Ten-pound weight gain over the past 3 months.
  – Mother died 2 months ago; depressed since then. Sleeping poorly.
  – Cough for 1 week, productive of yellow phlegm. No fevers. No hemoptysis. No wheezing. **Had two teeth pulled and was treated for a dental abscess 6 weeks ago**.

Discussion of Case 1

This is a straightforward case of accelerated angina, with typical risk factors and many classic features. The intermittent black stools and family history of colon cancer are potentially pertinent positives because anemia can lower the threshold for angina and could be a major contributing factor. If the patient had significant new anemia, the possible melena and family history of colon cancer would need to be presented in the HPI. The recent dental extractions and abscess are potentially relevant, since chest pain and cough are common symptoms of endocarditis; however, the absence of fever (a pertinent negative here) and the classic anginal features of the chest pain make the diagnosis of endocarditis very unlikely. The melena, family history of colon cancer, and recent dental abscess might be thought of as *conditional* or *potential* positives, which become relevant only in certain circumstances – if the hemoglobin had dropped from 14 to 7 over the past 6 months, say, or if the patient began spiking fevers after admission and had positive blood cultures.

Note that pertinent positives are most useful in making a prima facie ("at first glance" or "on the face of it") argument for a given diagnosis. Pertinent positives alone are less helpful when it comes to generating a differential and working through the various diagnostic possibilities. Pertinent positives mostly *rule in*; pertinent negatives mostly *rule out*. Thus it is not enough to have a diagnosis that is strongly supported by pertinent positives alone; competing diagnoses will need to be ruled out with pertinent negatives. Consider a more challenging case of chest pain where pertinent negatives take the differential in an unexpected direction, and one obscure but key pertinent positive helps to confirm the unusual diagnosis (in the case description, pertinent positives will be given in bold print, pertinent negatives in italics).

Case 2: Chest Pain

A *43-year-old* Hispanic man with a history of asthma and **hyperlipidemia** presented with 10 days of **substernal chest pain, initially with moderate exertion, but occurring at rest for the past day**. The chest pain is "**tight and squeezing**" in character, **radiates to the neck**, and is *not pleuritic*. It is associated with **shortness of breath, nausea, and diaphoresis**. It was **relieved with rest until today**; it is *not relieved with food or antacids*. He has *no history of hypertension or diabetes and has never smoked. There is no family history of heart disease.*

Past medical history: Mild-intermittent asthma, gets occasional wheezing with heavy exertion only (less than twice a week). No asthma hospitalizations. **Hyperlipidemia, on simvastatin**; recent **LDL cholesterol was 128**, *HDL was 56*.

- Medications: Simvastatin, albuterol inhaler as needed.
- Past surgical history: Remote appendectomy and left knee arthroscopy.
- Family history: Father 69, treated for HTN. Mother died at 42 of ovarian cancer. Two healthy sisters.
- Social history: Non-smoker, no current illicit drug use. Drinks two to three beers several days per week. *Last cocaine use was 19 years ago.* Works in a foundry; married with no children.
- Sexual history: Monogamous with his spouse for 15 years; no history of sex with men. **Treated for an STD in Guatemala 20 years ago; unsure of diagnosis, treated with "pills."**
- Review of systems:

  - Chronic low back pain.
  - GERD symptoms two to three times per week.
  - Mild psoriasis, uses topical steroid cream as needed.
  - *No leg claudication symptoms.*

- Pertinent PE findings:

  - Normal vital signs, BP 132/74.
  - *No carotid, abdominal, or femoral bruits.*
  - JVP 7 cm.
  - Lungs clear.
  - Heart regular S1S2, no murmur or gallop.
  - *Normal femoral, DP, and PT pulses.*
  - No peripheral edema.

- Electrocardiogram: Normal sinus rhythm, **variable ST depression in anterior and inferior leads on serial ECGs.**
- Left heart catheterization results: **98% ostial stenosis of left main, 70% ostial stenosis of RCA**; *coronary arteries otherwise clear.*

Discussion of Case 2

As in the first case, the pertinent positives in Case 2 strongly support a diagnosis of accelerated angina. The pertinent negatives, however, do not point to atherosclerosis as the cause of the angina. The patient is young and has very few cardiac risk factors and no family history. His hyperlipidemia is controlled with simvastatin. There are no signs or symptoms of peripheral vascular disease, which often accompanies coronary artery disease. Most striking is the severe ostial disease in the left main and RCA with *no distal coronary disease at all.* This suggests that the pathology is in the aorta, not the coronary arteries. The differential diagnosis for aortitis with coronary ostial involvement includes giant cell arteritis, Takayasu arteritis, and syphilis [1]. Giant cell arteritis occurs in patients over 50 and generally presents with tongue or jaw claudication and/or loss of vision; isolated coronary ostial disease would be extremely rare. Takayasu arteritis typically occurs in young women and manifests as ocular ischemic syndromes, stroke, arm ischemia ("pulseless disease"), or severe hypertension, depending on which aortic branches are affected. Syphilitic aortitis, on the other hand, does present as isolated coronary ostial stenosis, and the patient's history of an STD 20 years ago with uncertain treatment is a key pertinent positive that supports this diagnosis, which was subsequently confirmed with a positive RPR at 1:64 and positive MHA-TP. Syphilitic aortitis with coronary ostial stenosis generally requires coronary artery bypass surgery. The surgery is usually done before antibiotics are given because of the theoretical risk of fatal ostial occlusion due to the Jarisch-Herxheimer reaction, a systemic inflammatory response that can occur with penicillin treatment. This patient had a lumbar puncture to rule out neurosyphilis and then successful coronary artery bypass surgery followed by treatment with 14 days of IV penicillin.

In the case discussed above, the pertinent negatives are critical in determining the true cause and anatomic location of the problem. In the following case of abdominal pain, one key pertinent negative alters our take on the case:

Case 3: Abdominal Pain

An 82-year-old woman with history of HTN, type 2 DM, COPD, gout, and remote diverticulitis presents with 3 days of **right upper quadrant abdominal pain**, **nausea**, and **vomiting**, with **fever to 101°** since last night. The pain is **colicky** and **radiates to a point just below the right scapula**. The pain **awakened her** last night. Nothing relieves the pain; it seems to be **aggravated when she eats fatty foods**. She has had **three to four similar but milder episodes of RUQ pain over the past year**. There is *no constipation, diarrhea, melena, hematochezia, or GERD symptoms. No hematuria, dysuria, or flank pain*. She takes an 81-mg aspirin daily, but *no NSAIDs*. She was hospitalized 7 years ago for uncomplicated acute diverticulitis, which resolved with antibiotic treatment.

- Medications: Aspirin, atorvastatin, lisinopril, amlodipine, allopurinol, glargine insulin, and aspart insulin.
- Past surgical history: *Appendectomy 45 years ago; total abdominal hysterectomy 34 years ago.*
- Family history: Mother died of lung cancer at age 69; father died of a CVA at age 57.
- Social history: No alcohol, tobacco, or illicit drug use. Retired university professor. Married, no children.
- Review of systems:
  - Glycemic control has been good with recent fasting glucoses 90s to 140s, random glucoses <180, and no hypoglycemic symptoms. Last HA1c was 7.6%.
  - No chest pain.
  - Mild wheezing two to three times per week, relieved with prn albuterol inhaler. SOB with walking 100 yards or climbing one flight of stairs.
  - Chronic arthritis pain in the left knee; chronic low back pain, stable.

- Pertinent PE findings:
  - Vital signs **101.8110 24 96/64**
  - *Sclera anicteric.*
  - Lungs clear.
  - Heart regular S1S2 no murmur of gallop
  - Abdomen with decreased bowel sounds; **moderate RUQ tenderness with Murphy sign present**; *no masses, no organomegaly.*
- Pertinent lab and imaging results: **WBC 16,800 with left shift**; *liver function tests normal.*
- Right upper quadrant ultrasound: *No gallstones; no gallbladder wall thickening or pericholecystic fluid.*

Discussion of Case 3

This is an elderly patient with classic signs and symptoms of acute cholecystitis. Surprisingly, her RUQ ultrasound shows no gallstones and no other findings to suggest cholecystitis – a highly pertinent negative. We might want to look for a source of fever outside the biliary tract, but it's hard to ignore the many positive findings that make a very compelling case for cholecystitis. The key here is not to abandon the diagnosis of cholecystitis in the face of a negative ultrasound but to consider a more unusual possibility: acalculous cholecystitis. Acalculous cholecystitis usually occurs in very sick ICU patients with such conditions as shock, sepsis, trauma, burns, and prolonged TPN. It is associated with increased mortality, often from gangrenous cholecystitis complicated by perforation and peritonitis. The sensitivity of ultrasound in acalculous cholecystitis (criteria include gallbladder wall thickening >3.5 mm, pericholecystic fluid, and sludge) ranges widely from 29% to 92% [2], so the possibility of a false negative RUQ ultrasound must always be considered. In a patient with signs and symptoms of cholecystitis and a negative or equivocal ultrasound, HIDA radionuclide cholescintigraphy is a reasonable next step to rule out acalculous cholecystitis. This patient had a positive HIDA scan with non-visualization of the gallbladder and was treated successfully with IV antibiotics followed by laparoscopic cholecystectomy.

In some cases, patients present with overlapping sets of pertinent positives that seem to suggest more than one diagnosis. Consider the case of a woman with chronic headache and worsening symptoms for the past 3 months:

Case 4: Chronic Headache

A 34-year-old woman with a history of chronic headache since age 17 presents with worsening headache symptoms. **Previously the headaches were moderate in severity and occurred once or twice a week; for the past 3 months, she has had severe daily headaches.** The headaches generally **occur late in the day** and **start with neck and occipital pain and then become throbbing and bifrontal**. They **last up to 3–4 h**, sometimes longer. The headaches are associated with **photophobia and phonophobia.** There is *no associated aura, photoscotomata, neck stiffness, weakness, paresthesias, lacrimation, rhinorrhea, temporal tenderness, or loss of vision.* **Until 3 months ago, naproxen 400 mg gave prompt relief**, but it has been **less effective recently despite taking it two or three times daily**. She has *tried sumatriptan several times in the past without relief.* The *headaches do not seem to correlate with her menstrual cycle; she does not take oral contraceptives.* **Lying still in a dark, quiet room is sometimes helpful**, but she often gets headaches at work and cannot find a place to lie down. Her **stress level at work and in her personal life has been high recently**.

- Past medical history: Chronic headache, seasonal allergic rhinitis, obesity (BMI 34.2).
- Medications: Naproxen as above, loratadine 10 mg daily.
- Family history: **Mother had surgical repair of a brain aneurysm at age 56**. Father, 62, has hypertension. Two younger sisters and one brother, all in good health. No children.

- Social history: **Smoker, one pack per day for 17 years.** Alcohol, one to two drinks per month. No illicit drug use. Sexually active with one partner, who usually uses a condom. Works as a sales manager, travels frequently.
- Review of systems:
  - Eczema of hands and wrists, uses a topical steroid as needed.

- Pertinent PE findings:
  - Vital signs 98.4 76 14,118/78
  - *Normal fundoscopic exam; optic discs are sharp.*
  - Ears normal. *No sinus tenderness.* Oropharynx normal.
  - *No temporal tenderness;* **mild occipital and cervical paraspinous tenderness.**
  - *Normal neck flexion, extension, and rotation without pain.*
  - *Cranial nerves II–XII normal; DTRs, motor, and sensory exam globally normal.*

Discussion of Case 4

This patient has symptoms of both tension and migraine headaches and does not fit neatly into either category. Tension headaches typically occur later in the day, start in the neck and occipital area, and are usually relieved with simple analgesics such as naproxen. Migraine headaches are associated with photophobia and phonophobia and are often eased by lying in a dark, quiet room; migraines are usually hemifrontal rather than bifrontal and are more likely to respond to triptans than NSAIDs. This patient probably has mixed headache syndrome, with both tension and migraine features. The worsening of her headaches over the past 3 months is associated with multiple daily doses of naproxen, which raises the possibility of medication overuse headache (also known as analgesic-induced headache or "rebound headache"). The International Headache Society diagnostic criteria for medication overuse headache are as follows:

- Headache present on >15 days/month.
- Regular overuse for >3 months of one or more drugs that can be taken for acute and/or symptomatic treatment of headache.
- Headache has developed or markedly worsened during medication overuse [3].

Treatment for medication overuse headache requires withdrawal of the offending medication, usually with initiation of a prophylactic headache medicine either immediately or after a period of detoxification [4].

In this case, the pertinent positives and negatives direct us to the primary diagnosis of mixed headache, and the timeline of recent events – the worsening daily headaches and excessive use of naproxen over 3 months – leads to the secondary diagnosis of medication overuse headache.

The Dog that Didn't Bark

In a perfect world, all patients would present with classic signs and symptoms and carry a clear-cut diagnosis. In the real world, unfortunately, this is not so. Patients present with atypical symptoms, ambiguous findings, and *formes frustes* instead of textbook illnesses. "Do not expect to find a perfect set of symptoms, signs and tests characterizing a given condition in order to make a diagnosis," writes Ami Schattner. "Any combination may occur and sometimes even a single symptom and sign may suggest the correct diagnosis" [5]. But which symptom or sign is it? Which pertinent positive or negative is the key finding? It might be the most obvious suspect, but what about "the curious incident of the dog in the night-time?" The curious incident was that the dog didn't bark, Sherlock Holmes informs us, because he knew the midnight intruder [6]. This is perhaps our best-known (and most beloved) literary example of the pertinent negative. Keep it in mind as you work through a complex case. What is inconsistent or out of place? What is missing? Consider the chest x-ray (Fig. 5.1) of a 75-year-old woman with a long history of dysphagia and wheezing.

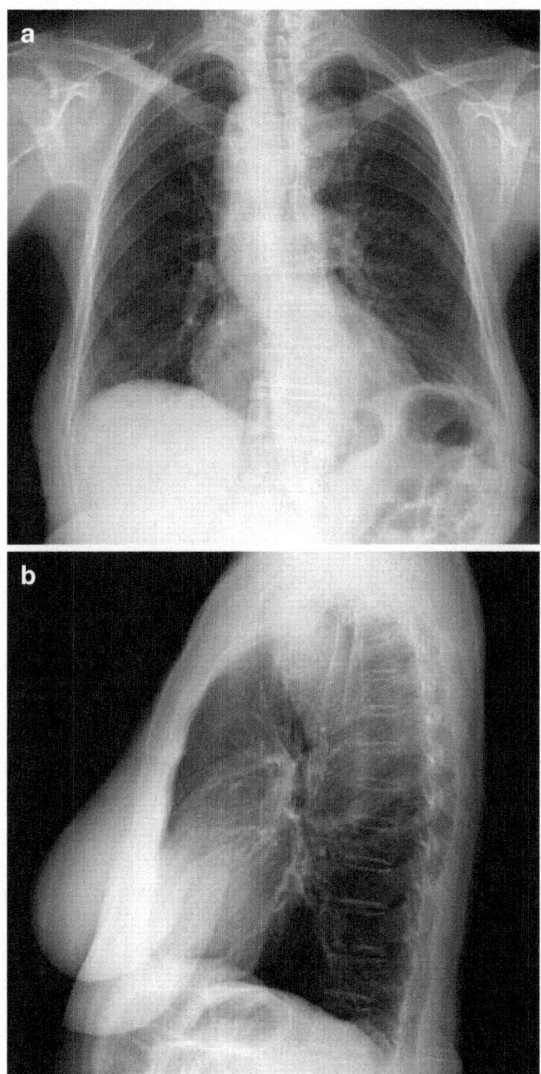

FIGURE 5.1 Chest radiographs. (a) Posteroanterior view showing right-sided aortic arch and abnormal bilateral paratracheal stripes. (b) Lateral view showing a superomedial mediastinal mass displacing the trachea forward. (Reproduced from Carbone et al. [7], Copyright 2008, with permission from BMJ Publishing Group Ltd.)

In this case, the key finding is the anomalous right-sided location of the aortic arch and descending aorta, which occurs in about 0.1% of patients. This is sometimes associated with a Kommerell's diverticulum, which refers to the bulbous configuration of the origin of an aberrant left subclavian artery in the setting of a right-sided aortic arch. Kommerell's diverticulum is thought to be an embryologic remnant of the fourth dorsal aortic arch. It can produce a mass-like effect on the esophagus and trachea, which caused the symptoms in this patient [7]. Surgical treatment options include a hybrid approach with midline sternotomy for arch debranching, followed by endovascular repair of the aneurysm [8].

Pertinent Positives and Negatives: Six Suggestions

1. In your oral presentation, begin with the timeline for the chief complaint and then use the pertinent positives and negatives to bring the diagnosis into focus.
2. Learn and memorize the pertinent positives for common illnesses. These must be presented in the HPI and can be used to make a prima facie case for a diagnosis.
3. Based on your initial differential diagnosis, create a list of pertinent negatives for your case presentation. A comprehensive list of pertinent negatives shows that you have considered a broad differential, while at the same time narrowing it and making an argument for the most likely diagnosis.
4. Be an active listener on rounds. Every case presentation will include pertinent positives and negatives, and you can learn a great deal from listening and thinking about the differential diagnosis as others present. Also listen very carefully to the attending physician's comments and requests for further information.
5. Get involved in case discussions. Pertinent positives and negatives are the currency of these conversations.

6. See and admit as many patients as possible. Repetition is extremely important in medicine. For any disease, there are as many unique presentations as there are patients. Diagnosis largely depends on recognizing these variations on a theme. Careful consideration of pertinent positives and negatives will help you to recognize the underlying patterns and possibilities in patients with atypical presentations.

References

1. Tavora F, Burke A. Review of isolated ascending aortitis: differential diagnosis, including syphilitic, Takayasu's and giant cell aortitis. Pathology. 2006;38(4):302–8.
2. Huffman JL, Schenker S. Acute acalculous cholecystitis: a review. Clin Gastroenterol Hepatol. 2010;8(1):15–22.
3. Headache Classification Committee of the International Headache Society (IHS). The international classification of headache disorders, 3rd edition. Cephalalgia. 2018;38(1):1–211.
4. Kristofferson ES, Lundqvist C. Medication-overuse headache: epidemiology, diagnosis and treatment. Ther Adv Drug Saf. 2014;5(2):87–99.
5. Schattner A. Teaching clinical medicine: the key principals. QJM. 2015;108(6):435–42.
6. Conan Doyle A, Blaze S. The complete Sherlock Holmes. New York: Doubleday; 1930. p. 335–50.
7. Carbone I, Sedati P, Galea N, Algeri E, Passariello R. Right-sided aortic arch with Kommerell's diverticulum: 64-DCTA with 3D reconstructions. Thorax. 2008;63(7):662.
8. Knepper J, Criado E. Surgical treatment of Kommerell's diverticulum and other saccular arch aneurysms. J Vasc Surg. 2013;57(4):951–4.

Chapter 6
The Diagnostic Power of Description

The Art of Description

The oral presentation is the place to show your descriptive powers. Your patient's key symptoms and physical exam findings should be thoroughly and lavishly described. Think of the way a lepidopterist would describe the features of a gorgeous blue morpho butterfly or of how an eloquent mechanic might expound on the contours of his 1962 Corvette and its 327 cc engine. These things are lingeringly and lovingly described, with a level of detail and pitch of fervor that would entrance even a casual listener. This is the kind of performance you should aim for on morning rounds.

This is not just to show that you're a brilliant medical student, although it certainly doesn't hurt. Careful and detailed description serves an essential function in the process of diagnosis. Consider William Osler's 1887 description of the auscultation findings in a 25-year-old man who had fallen and pierced his left axilla with a lead pencil several years before:

> The heart sounds are clear at apex and base. There is no special accentuation of the aortic second sound; no murmur in the right carotid, or in the right subclavian arteries. Over the outer half of the left infraclavicular area, on the corresponding portion of the clavicle, over the lower cervical triangle from the sterno-mastoid border to the attachment of the trapezius there is a loud continuous bruit. This murmur is also heard with great intensity in the axilla, down the inner surface of the arm, and on the front and

© Springer Nature Switzerland AG 2019
C. D. Packer, *Presenting Your Case*,
https://doi.org/10.1007/978-3-030-13792-2_6

back of the fore-arm. It is very loud and distinct in the palm of the
hand and in the finger tips.... At one point only, just below the
clavicle, there is a slight systolic intensification of the murmur.
Posteriorly the murmur is heard in the subscapular space and
feebly upon the scapula.... Pressure upon the axillary artery high
up in the arm-pit caused complete disappearance of the thrill and
the murmur in the clavicular region. The diagnosis of arteriovenous aneurysm was made. [1]

Osler's meticulous description of the auscultation findings,
including the response to compression of the axillary artery,
clinches the diagnosis of a rare axillary arteriovenous aneurysm. Remember that this case report was written decades
before the development of diagnostic angiography and ultra-
sonography. In the nineteenth century, physicians had to rely
entirely on the accuracy of their physical examination findings, and their only gold standard was the autopsy. As another
example, Walter Broadbent published four cases of chronic
pericarditis in 1895, "in each of which there is visible retraction, synchronous with the cardiac systole, of the left back in
the region of the eleventh and twelfth ribs, and in three of
which there is also systolic retraction of less degree in the
same region of the right back." He goes on to give his reasoning to support the diagnosis of adherent pericardium:

The only means of causing this retraction on both sides seems to
be the diaphragm, which, if pulled upon, would have more effect
on the floating eleventh and twelfth ribs than on the fixed ones.
In cases of large heart with adherent pericardium there is a considerable area of the ventricles closely adherent to the central
tendon of the diaphragm, and the powerful contraction of the
hypertrophied heart must give a decided tug to this structure. [2]

These are examples of descriptions so clear, detailed, and
accurate that they could be held up as archetypes of their
respective diseases (see also Sydenham's classic description
of measles in Chap. 4). Note that in both cases the description
led directly to the diagnosis.

But today's medical student might ask: why bother? (In
fact, one bold student did ask me this question during a
teaching session on cardiac auscultation). We have ultraso-
nography and echocardiography and a vast array of other
imaging modalities that Osler and Broadbent could hardly

have imagined. Who cares any more about the physical exam, when we have the tools to make a definitive diagnosis at any time? It is true, unfortunately, that physical exam skills have dropped off alarmingly in our students and younger practitioners [3]. "Despite the abundance of auscultatory findings with direct clinical rather than esoteric relevance," write Alam et al., "the requirement for demonstrating an adequate level of competence when performing cardiac auscultation has fallen to unbelievably low levels" [4]. Why does it matter? If the physical exam is inaccurate, the working diagnosis will probably be erroneous, and the wrong test – or no test – will be ordered, and important diagnostic findings will be missed or misinterpreted. Varghese et al. have shown that inadequacies of the physical examination can be "a major contributor to missed or delayed diagnosis, unnecessary exposure to contrast and radiation, incorrect treatment, and other adverse consequences" [5]. In addition, a slapdash approach to physical diagnosis can lead to wasteful over-testing. In a study of 3462 children in Fiji who were screened for rheumatic heart disease, 349 were found to have a murmur, yet only 29 (8.7%) of these patients had an abnormality confirmed on echocardiography [6]. This suggests that many children with innocent murmurs and (very likely) normal heart sounds were referred for echocardiography, at significant inconvenience and expense.

Another consequence of the decline in physical exam skills seems to be a generational drop-off in our students' descriptive powers. Superficial examinations do not lead to lush descriptions. Unfortunately, we seem to be ceding our clinical description to radiologists, who dwell in Plato's Cave and deal with shadows of reality.

Diagnosis Through Description

Medical students can make a difference for their patients in many ways. They can be interpreters, advocates, and good listeners; they can soothe pain and ease anxiety. But students can also serve their patients simply by giving clear, accurate, and appropriately detailed descriptions of the key history and physical exam findings on rounds. For example, in the case of a patient admitted with shortness of breath and a new heart murmur, a typical student might describe the murmur only as "a systolic murmur at the right upper sternal border." While accurate as far as it goes, this is a woefully inadequate description of what is probably the most important clue in the case. We need rich and elaborate descriptions of these key physical findings! The history suggests a diagnosis, and – very frequently – the accurate and thorough physical exam confirms it. Here is a superb student's dynamic description of the same systolic murmur:

> The rhythm is regular with a diminished second heart sound and no audible S2 splitting. There is a 3/6 harsh, late systolic ejection murmur, loudest at the right upper sternal border and also audible at the left lower sternal border. It decreases with the Valsalva maneuver, and returns to full intensity 5-6 beats after release of Valsalva. The carotid pulses are weak and slow-rising, and there is a pulse delay with the radial pulse occurring after S2.

These are classic findings of severe aortic stenosis. An echocardiogram reveals that the aortic valve area is critically low at 0.6 cm^2, and the patient is taken for urgent aortic valve replacement. In this case, the student's methodical physical exam has revealed the diagnosis and helped to expedite treatment for a sick patient. Would this patient have gotten an echocardiogram anyway? Perhaps, but the student's convincing description of critical aortic stenosis expedited the diagnosis and got the patient to the operating room sooner rather than later.

Consider the case of a 67-year-old man with a new complaint of leg pain that has been limiting his activity. The pedestrian student history might go as follows:

> For the past 3 months, he has been getting pain in both legs whenever he walks about a half block. The pain is relieved with rest.

The more thoughtful student, who has spent a little more time teasing out the symptoms with his patient, might give the following description:

For the past 3 months, he has been getting pain and numbness in both buttocks and posterior thighs whenever he walks about a half block. The pain is relieved only if he stops walking and then sits down; if he continues to stand, the pain persists. He has noticed the same pain when he stands for 10 minutes to do the dishes, or if he stands to wait for the bus. Again, the pain is relieved promptly when he sits down.

Taken at face value, the first student's story sounds like intermittent claudication – exertional pain due to arterial insufficiency in the legs. The history obtained by the second student, however, strongly supports a diagnosis of pseudo-claudication due to lumbar spinal stenosis (Table 6.1). The distinction between claudication and pseudoclaudication is important, because the diagnostic work-up and treatment are completely different: ankle-brachial indices, angiography, and vascular stenting or bypass for claudication, versus lumbar MRI, physical therapy, and (if necessary) lumbar decompression

TABLE 6.1 Claudication vs. pseudoclaudication

	Claudication	Pseudoclaudication
Characteristic of discomfort	Cramping, tightness, aching, fatigue	Same as claudication plus tingling, burning, numbness
Location of discomfort	Buttock, hip, thigh, calf, foot	Same as claudication
Unilateral vs. bilateral	Often unilateral	Bilateral
Exercise-induced	Yes	Variable
Distance	Consistent	Variable
Occurs with standing	No	Yes
Action for relief	Stop walking, stand still	Sit or lean forward
Time to relief	<5 min	≤30 min

surgery for pseudoclaudication. An incorrect initial diagnosis could lead to wasteful testing and delayed treatment.

Medical students tend to worry about the words they use to describe their findings. They are concerned that their descriptions are not sufficiently "medical" or "technical" and strive to find a vocabulary that conforms to the expectations of their teachers. Georges Bordage has pointed out the importance of semantic qualifiers (essentially "useful adjectives" such as unilateral, bilateral, constant, throbbing, acute, monarticular, etc.) that allow the listening clinician to recognize the "prototype" of the disease [7]. Bordage suggests that students must learn to "translate" their case descriptions into these useful terms, which I think occurs naturally as students begin to pick up the descriptive vocabulary of their more experienced co-workers in the hospital or clinic. Use these descriptors, but by all means, go beyond them when the situation demands a more creative approach. The icepick headache, the sandpaper rash of scarlet fever, and the *peau d'orange* skin changes of inflammatory breast cancer all stick in our memories because they are creative, unexpected, and perfectly apt descriptions of illness.

More Examples: Sketchy Depictions Versus Deep Descriptions

Consider the following examples of key findings from the history and physical exam as presented first by an average student, and then by a student who understands the importance of deep description. Note the diagnostic power of the more nuanced descriptions.

Knee Pain

The patient has had right knee pain for 6 months. It hurts more with weight bearing and sometimes swells up. He does not recall any injury. On exam, there is no warmth or effusion, and the range of motion is normal (*Diagnosis: Knee pain*).

The patient has had right knee pain for 6 months. It hurts more with walking and stair-climbing and swells up occasionally when he is very active. There is no instability, but the joint sometimes locks and bending it becomes very painful. On exam, there is tenderness at the medial joint line; no warmth or effusion. There is no medial or lateral laxity, and the anterior and posterior drawer signs are negative. The McMurray sign is positive (there is a painful click with simultaneous extension and internal rotation of the lower leg) (*Diagnosis: Medial meniscal tear*).

Hip Pain

The patient complains of left hip pain for the past 3 weeks. It occurs with walking or prolonged sitting. It improves temporarily when she takes ibuprofen. On exam, there is normal range of motion in the left hip and no warmth or swelling (*Diagnosis: Hip pain*).

The patient complains of left hip pain for the past 3 weeks. There is moderate discomfort in the lateral hip with walking and prolonged sitting. There is significant pain when she lies on her left side at night. Ibuprofen gives temporary relief. On exam, there is marked tenderness over the left greater trochanter. Internal and external rotations are normal, with no pain (*Diagnosis: Left trochanteric bursitis*).

Prostate Symptoms

The patient complains of 2 months of dribbling, slow stream, and incomplete emptying. He gets up to urinate three times per night. There is no dysuria or hematuria. On rectal exam, the prostate is moderately enlarged (*Diagnosis: BPH*).

The patient complains of 2 months of urinary frequency, urgency, slow stream, incomplete emptying, and nocturia × 3. The onset of symptoms was abrupt. There is no dysuria or hematuria. He also has pain with ejaculation. On rectal exam, the prostate is moderately enlarged, boggy, and extremely tender (*Diagnosis: Chronic prostatitis*).

Groin Pain and Bulging

The patient complains of right groin pain, pressure, and bulging for the past 3–4 weeks. It is worse when he lifts heavy objects at work or strains to have a bowel movement. On exam, there is no inguinal hernia; there is mild right scrotal fullness and tenderness (*Diagnosis: Groin pain, hydrocele*).

The patient complains of right groin pain, pressure, and bulging for the past 3–4 weeks. It is worse when he lifts heavy objects at work or strains to have a bowel movement. No nausea, vomiting, or abdominal distention. On exam, there is no direct inguinal hernia. In the scrotum, there is a large, tender, non-reducible mass that passes through the right inguinal ring; the mass does not transilluminate; bowel sounds are audible in the scrotum (*Diagnosis: Indirect inguinal hernia*).

Rash

The patient complains of 5 days of low-grade fevers, chills, headache, and joint pains. Two days ago she noticed a red spot on her right thigh, which she attributes to a spider bite. On exam, there is a 5 × 5 cm erythematous patch on the right thigh with a small central eschar (*Diagnosis: Viral syndrome, spider bite*).

The patient complains of 5 days of low-grade fevers, chills, headache, and joint pains. Seven days ago she went hiking in the woods and walked through bushes and tall grass in short pants. Two days ago, she noticed a red circular rash on her right anterior thigh, which has increased in size. She does not recall seeing any ticks on her leg; she thinks she might have had a spider bite on the leg while she was sleeping. On exam, there is a 5 × 5 cm erythematous, macular, target-shaped rash on the right anterior thigh with a small central eschar (*Diagnosis: Lyme disease with erythema migrans*).

"Well, of course," a student might say on reading this chapter. "It's important to take a thorough history and do a good exam. That's obvious." Yes, very true, but we're also talking here about presenting your case effectively and convincingly. In my experience, students commonly give too much detail about normal or marginally significant physical findings, and not enough detail about the critical parts of the exam. And sometimes, even if they do focus clearly on the key findings, their descriptions lack the depth and conviction required to make a strong argument for the diagnosis. *Focus on the key findings, and describe them with passion and precision.* This is the mantra for the oral case presentation.

References

1. Osler W. William Osler: original papers 1881–1897. In: Works of Sir William Osler. http://digitalcommons.library.tmc.edu/osler/1. Accessed 26 Jul 2018.
2. Broadbent W. An unpublished physical sign. Lancet. 1895;2:200.
3. Sandeep J. The demise of the physical exam. N Engl J Med. 2006;354:548–51.
4. Alam U, Asghar O, Khan SQ, Hayat S, Malik RA. Cardiac auscultation: an essential clinical skill in decline. Br J Cardiol. 2010;17:8–10.
5. Verghese A, Charlton B, Kassirer JP, Ramsey M, Ioannidis JP. Inadequacies of physical examination as a cause of medical errors and adverse events: a collection of vignettes. Am J Med. 2015;128(12):1322–4.
6. Steer AC, Kado J, Wilson N, Tuiketei T, Batzloff M, Waqatakirewa L, et al. High prevalence of rheumatic heart disease by clinical and echocardiographic screening among children in Fiji. J Heart Valve Dis. 2009;18:327–35.
7. Bordage G. Elaborated knowledge: a key to successful diagnostic thinking. Acad Med. 1994;69(11):883–5.

Chapter 7
The Assessment and Plan

Elements of the Assessment and Plan

The assessment and plan is the culmination of the oral case presentation. It consists of a brief summary of the case, a discussion of the differential diagnosis, an argument for the leading diagnosis, a diagnostic testing strategy, and a treatment plan (Table 7.1). A robust assessment and plan is the holy grail for third-year medical students. Those who can produce a broad differential diagnosis, narrow it, and make a coherent and convincing argument for the leading diagnosis will earn the praise and respect of their teachers. A concise and focused assessment also improves patient care because it filters out the "background noise" of the case and keeps the team on track.

An essential first step in making a strong assessment is to identify the key findings in the case. As noted in Chap. 2, collecting the key findings is a way to distil the case down to its basic elements in order to think about it, discuss it, and formulate a differential diagnosis. The key findings can be drawn from any and all parts of the history, the physical exam, the initial lab testing and imaging results, and the response (or lack of response) to treatment. For example, the key findings in a patient with acute decompensated heart failure might be dyspnea, orthopnea, weight gain, hypoxemia, pulmonary rales, JVP of 14 cm, leg edema, Pro-BNP of 3500, and Kerley B lines on chest x-ray. Key findings for a

C. D. Packer, *Presenting Your Case*,
https://doi.org/10.1007/978-3-030-13792-2_7

TABLE 7.1 Elements of the assessment and plan

Elements of the assessment and plan	Comments
Brief case summary	Summarize key findings from the history, physical exam, lab testing, and imaging
Differential diagnosis	Use the key findings to develop a differential diagnosis
	Start with a broad differential, then narrow
Argument for the leading diagnosis	Make a persuasive argument for the leading diagnosis or diagnoses
	Explain why alternative diagnoses are less likely
Diagnostic testing strategy	Specific tests to rule in or rule out
	Show understanding of test characteristics and Bayesian reasoning
Treatment plan	Medications, IV fluids, nursing protocols, etc.
	Incorporate high-value care principles

patient with acute hepatitis might include recent consumption of questionable oysters, malaise, fever, scleral icterus, RUQ tenderness with hepatomegaly, transaminase and bilirubin elevations, and a positive anti-HAV IgM. In these two cases, the key findings steer us to an obvious diagnosis. Sometimes, however, the key findings are indecipherable at first glance. When a patient presents with fever, migratory polyarthritis, lymphadenopathy, episcleritis, abnormal liver function tests, and a nodular rash, the diagnosis is unclear and differential diagnosis is difficult. We'll discuss the nuts and bolts of differential diagnosis in Chap. 8. For now, let's assume that you have already thought through the differential, and focus instead on how to deliver an effective assessment and an actionable plan.

Let Us Know What You're Thinking

The assessment is all about explaining your reasoning and making an argument for what you think is the likeliest diagnosis. How you structure the assessment is less important than just getting your thoughts out there. As an attending, the most satisfying part of my day (other than seeing a patient get better) is when a student makes a coherent and convincing argument for a diagnosis on rounds. One of the defining attributes of a physician is the capacity to make a diagnosis; to see a student reach that milestone is a wonderful thing.

Consider several examples of student assessments presented in different styles, emphasizing a variety of diagnostic questions and conundrums. The common feature of these assessments is that they give the reasoning that leads to the proposed diagnosis. Note that the assessments are very specific, focused, and granular. Generalities about asthma or cirrhosis are fine for teaching sessions, but the assessment should get right down to the business of sorting out the differential diagnosis and making a treatment plan.

I have included references for articles that the students might have used to prepare their presentations and back up their arguments:

1. Mrs. Brown is a 52-year-old woman who has been hospitalized twice for treatment-resistant asthma since her initial hospitalization last month for an opioid overdose with respiratory failure. She was prescribed an albuterol inhaler, but it hasn't been effective. The odd thing is that she's persistently short of breath, even at rest, but I don't hear any wheezing in the lungs. I do hear some inspiratory stridor over the upper airways. The differential diagnosis for stridor includes bilateral vocal cord paralysis, foreign body, epiglottitis, and tracheal stenosis. She does not have neurologic conditions or symptoms of a viral infection such as EBV that might cause vocal cord paralysis; there is no history to suggest a foreign body. Patients with epiglottitis

usually have high fever, sore throat, and difficulty swallowing; our patient has none of those symptoms and does not look toxic. As for tracheal stenosis, she was emergently intubated last month when she had the opioid overdose, and tracheal stenosis can be a complication of traumatic intubation [1, 2]. I think tracheal stenosis is a strong possibility. An ENT consult would be helpful.

2. Ms. Hessler is a 52-year-old woman with Child C alcoholic cirrhosis who was admitted for worsening ascites and shortness of breath. She was found to have a large right pleural effusion, which was tapped and determined to be transudative. The differential diagnosis for a transudative effusion includes heart failure, nephrotic syndrome, hepatic hydrothorax, and rare causes such as superior vena cava obstruction, constrictive pericarditis, and urinothorax [3]. Pleural effusions from heart failure are typically bilateral, but when they are unilateral, they are usually right-sided [4]. Hepatic hydrothorax (Fig. 7.1) occurs in 5–10% of patients with cirrhosis and is caused by leakage of ascites fluid into the thorax through a defect in the diaphragm [5]. It is usually right-sided; in one series of 77 patients with hepatic hydrothorax, 73% were right-sided, 17% were left-sided, and 10% were bilateral [6]. The patient has a very low albumin level due to her liver disease, but low albumin levels alone rarely cause pleural effusions [7]. I think the main question here is whether the transudative right-sided effusion is from heart failure or hepatic hydrothorax. Against heart failure, the jugular venous pressure is normal on exam, and the pro-BNP is not elevated. Real-time contrast-enhanced ultrasound [8] or nuclear imaging could confirm the diagnosis of hepatic hydrothorax.

3. Mr. Random is a 78-year-old man with hypertension, type 2 diabetes, and a non-ST elevation MI 3 months ago who came in last night with syncope. The syncope occurred with no warning while he was at rest in a seated position, and he regained alertness quickly with no confusion, tongue-biting, or incontinence. His initial ECG, head CT, and lab work-up were unremarkable. There were no clear precipitating

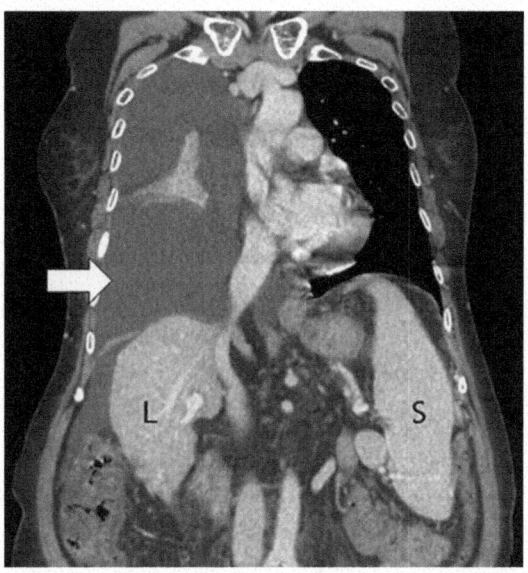

FIGURE 7.1 Hepatic hydrothorax. Coronal reformatted contrast-enhanced CT scan in a woman with liver cirrhosis showing gross right-sided pleural effusion (arrow). Also noted is presence of ascites, cirrhotic changes in liver (L), and splenomegaly (S). (Reprinted from Sureka et al. [5]. https://doi.org/10.1093/gastro/gov017 Gastroenterol Rep (Oxf) | © The Author(s) 2015. Published by Oxford University Press and the Digestive Science Publishing Co. Limited. This is an Open Access article distributed under the terms of the Creative Commons Attribution License (http://creativecommons.org/licenses/by/4.0/), which permits unrestricted reuse, distribution, and reproduction in any medium, provided the original work is properly cited)

factors for vasovagal syncope, such as dehydration, over-medication, or rapid position change. Seizure is unlikely with the normal head CT and absence of postictal confusion. He does not have risk factors for pulmonary embolism, and there was no pleuritic chest pain, leg swelling, dyspnea, tachycardia, or hypoxemia. It might have been a vasovagal episode, but I think we need to rule out an arrhythmia related to his coronary artery disease and recent

MI. We should monitor him on telemetry for 48 h and consider an event monitor, echocardiogram, and cardiology consult in case he needs an electrophysiologic study. If his ejection fraction is less than 35% on echocardiogram, he should have an implantable cardioverter-defibrillator (ICD) placed [9].

4. I'm not quite sure what to make of Ms. Coltman's chest pain. She's 53 and postmenopausal and has cardiac risk factors including hypertension, smoking, hyperlipidemia, and family history. Her chest pain is sharp, stabbing, and non-exertional, and she also complains of epigastric pain and nausea. Her ECG shows non-specific T-wave changes, and her troponin is negative. Although her chest pain is atypical, I'm concerned that she might have microvascular angina, which is common in postmenopausal women and has a 1.5-fold mortality risk compared to women without evidence of microvascular ischemia [10]. Rather than discharging her, I think she should have stress scintigraphy for functional assessment of the coronary arteries. If the stress test is consistent with microvascular ischemia (Fig. 7.2), she can be started on diltiazem and monitored for response.

5. Ms. Mayfield is a 69-year-old woman with stage III squamous cell lung cancer who was admitted with nausea, vomiting, and hyponatremia with a sodium of 122 mEq/L 3 days after completing a cycle of chemotherapy. She was drinking only water during the acute illness and was borderline orthostatic by pulse and blood pressure, with dry oral mucus membranes and skin tenting. Her urine sodium came back at <10 mEq/L. After hydration with IV normal saline overnight, her sodium level is up to 128 mEq/L and her orthostatic symptoms have resolved. Since she was hypovolemic with a low urine sodium on admission, and her serum sodium improved dramatically overnight with normal saline, I think that she has hypovolemic hyponatremia due to vomiting and dehydration. Mineralocorticoid deficiency is unlikely with a low urine sodium. Her low urine sodium, hypovolemic status, and response to normal saline are all inconsistent with SIADH. We should continue

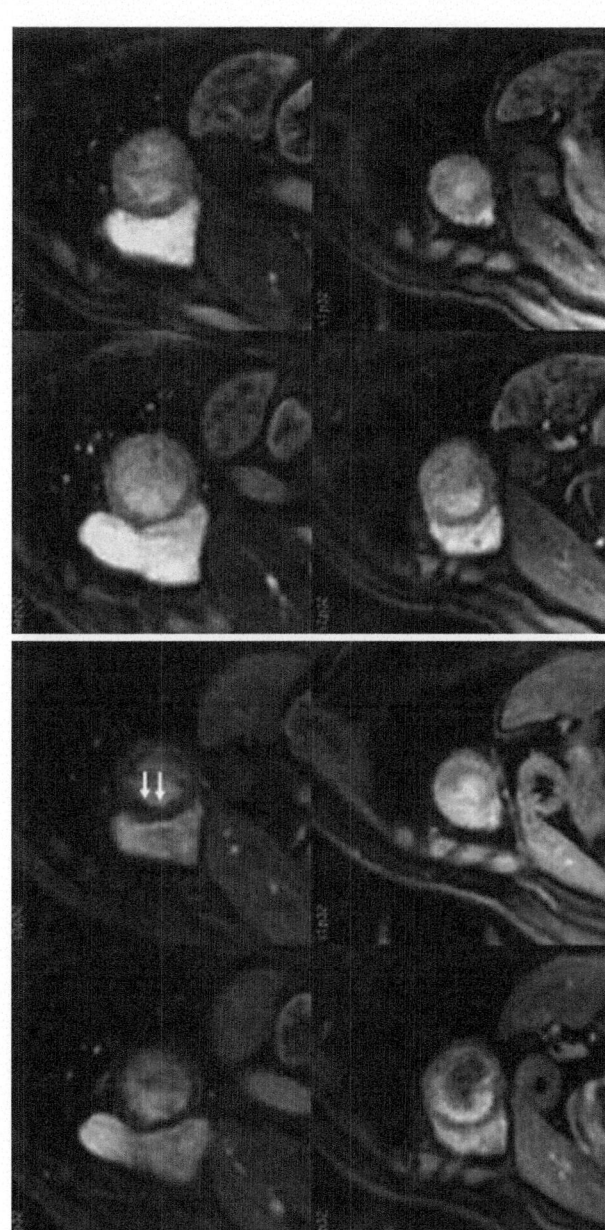

FIGURE 7.2 Cardiovascular perfusion magnetic resonance (CMR) first-pass study in a patient with microvascular ischemia (short-axis plane). In the left panels, obtained 26 s after administration of gadolinium at peak dobutamine stress test (DST), a perfusion defect is clearly visible in the mid-ventricular septum (arrows). The perfusion defect normalizes at rest (right). (Reprinted from Lanza et al. [22], Copyright 2008, with permission from Elsevier)

IV hydration with normal saline and supportive treatment
with antiemetics as needed [11].

6. Mr. Ryan is a 52-year-old man with hypertension who
comes to clinic today with 3 days of right leg pain and
swelling. He does not recall any injury, and there has been
no recent surgery, travel, or immobilization. Of note, he
was started on amlodipine 5 mg daily for hypertension
10 days ago. There is no personal or family history of blood
clots. On exam, there is mild calf tenderness on the right
with 1+ pitting pretibial edema, and trace pretibial edema
on the left. The right calf circumference is 1.5 cm larger
than the left. Amlodipine can cause leg swelling, but it's
usually bilateral, so further evaluation is needed. His Wells
Score is 1, which puts the pretest probability of DVT at
17%. Since the pretest probability is only moderate, we
should order a high-sensitivity D-dimer test. If the D-dimer
is negative, DVT is extremely unlikely, and we can hold off
on the leg ultrasound and send him home [12].

7. This is Mr. Corbo's third ER visit in 2 weeks for bilateral
shoulder pain and stiffness. He was diagnosed with a shoulder strain and treated with IM ketorolac the first time. At
his second visit, he had shoulder x-rays that showed mild
bilateral acromioclavicular and glenohumeral joint arthritis, and he was prescribed a course of naproxen, with no
improvement. Today his shoulders were so painful that he
needed help getting his shirt off for the exam. His ESR is
112 mm/h, and he has a mild normocytic anemia with hgb
11.0 g/dL. The pain is out of proportion to his mild arthritis,
and he has no signs of rotator cuff tears or tendinitis. The
bilateral symptoms suggest a systemic process. The high
ESR strongly supports a diagnosis of polymyalgia rheumatica. He doesn't have any visual symptoms, tongue or
jaw claudication, or temporal tenderness to suggest con-
current temporal arteritis. Late-onset rheumatoid arthritis
or other types of inflammatory arthritis are possible, but
the presentation would be atypical. At this point, I think we
should start prednisone 15 mg daily and monitor his

response; a rapid and dramatic response to low-dose corticosteroid treatment would clinch the diagnosis of PMR [13].

8. Ms. Larchmere is a 46-year-old woman with a history of multiple back surgeries and post-laminectomy syndrome, who was hospitalized for intractable back pain and then discharged to a rehab facility for intensive physical therapy. She was readmitted 3 days later with acute delirium, visual hallucinations, and a seizure. There was no lab or exam evidence of metabolic or infectious abnormalities. Head CT was negative, and EEG showed no focal abnormalities. There were no opioids or sedating medications, and a tox screen was negative. When we did her med reconciliation last night, we found that her baclofen (which she had been taking 20 mg TID for many years) had not been continued at the rehab facility. We searched the literature and found many case reports and case series describing a baclofen withdrawal syndrome that can involve agitation, insomnia, confusion, delusions, hallucinations, seizures, visual changes, psychosis, dyskinesia, hyperthermia, and increased spasticity [14, 15]. We restarted her baclofen, and she's substantially better this morning.

9. Mr. Hazel is a 24-year-old man with no known medical problems who was brought into the ER with lethargy and dysarthria after "drinking something" and then vomiting at a party late last night. He's tachycardic and tachypneic with Kussmaul breathing; his ABG reveals a metabolic acidosis, and his anion gap is very high at 42. The differential for an anion gap acidosis includes toxic ingestions, ketoacidosis, renal failure, and lactic acidosis. The glucose, creatinine, and lactate levels are normal, so DKA, lactic acidosis, and renal failure are ruled out. We've just gotten back his measured serum osmolality, and the osmolal gap is near-normal at 14. This does not rule out methanol or ethylene glycol toxicity, because the osmolal gap decreases and the anion gap rises over time after an ingestion due to the conversion of these alcohols to their toxic metabolites, formic acid and

oxalic acid (Fig. 7.3). Thus a patient who ingested methanol or ethylene glycol several hours ago could present with a high anion gap and a normal or near-normal osmolal gap [16]. Based on this possibility and the patient's history, we're still very concerned that this is a methanol or ethylene glycol ingestion. We've given the patient a dose of fomepizole and asked the nephrology team to see him for immediate dialysis. We're expecting methanol and ethylene glycol levels back from the lab momentarily; if these are negative, we'll need to reconsider the diagnosis. Alcoholic ketoacidosis (AKA) could cause a similar biochemical picture (anion gap metabolic acidosis with a modestly elevated osmolal gap) in a patient with binge drinking followed by 2–3 days of vomiting and dehydration, but it seems less likely because (1) we would not expect a change in mental status with AKA, and (2) it doesn't fit with the timeline we were given by friend who brought him in from the party. Treatment of AKA is simple: supportive treatment and aggressive hydration with D5 normal saline.

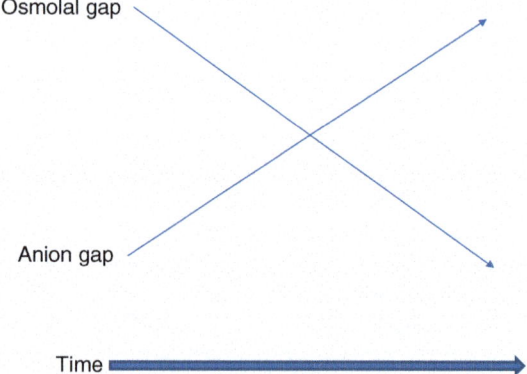

FIGURE 7.3 Changes in osmolal gap and anion gap over time in patients with toxic alcohol ingestions (methanol and ethylene glycol)

Assessment: Beyond Diagnosis

When admitting patients who already have a clear diagnosis, the focus of the assessment shifts to the treatment plan. This is the case for many night float and transfer admissions (see Chap. 3) as well as for patients who arrive from the ER or the clinic with an obvious and uncontroversial diagnosis. Therapy decisions for these patients can be just as complex and challenging as the most complicated diagnostic dilemmas:

1. Mrs. Kenilworth is a 69-year-old woman with widely metastatic breast cancer who has exhausted all treatment options. She comes in with worsening shortness of breath from her malignant pleural effusions and intractable pain. She seems ready to consider hospice care, but her two sons are adamant that "everything should be done for her," including intensive care, intubation, and electrical shock, despite our clear explanation as to why these measures would be uncomfortable, inhumane, and ultimately futile. I think we should have a family meeting and invite her oncologist and a member of the ethics committee to attend. I researched the question of medical futility and found that there are three central concepts:

   • Physicians are not obligated to provide treatments they believe are ineffective or harmful to patients.
   • Physicians should not initially just say "no" to patients concerning futile treatments but must engage in dialogue and discuss alternatives.
   • Physicians must always convey that medical *care is never* futile [17].

   I think that if we stress the benefits of palliative care – increased comfort, dignity, and peaceful surroundings – rather than focus on the negatives of futility and discomfort, there's a good chance that the patient and her sons will accept hospice care, which is clearly her best option at this point. We just need to listen to them and try to understand where they're coming from.

2. Mr. Morley is a 92-year-old man with hypertension, chronic atrial fibrillation, and "mild vascular dementia" who has been depressed since his wife died 2 months ago. Over the past month, he has had three ER visits and two hospitalizations for confusion and panic symptoms. He was evaluated by a psychiatrist and started on an antidepressant. He lives alone and wants to return to his apartment, but he was found to lack capacity, and we think he is unsafe to live alone at this point. His daughter is involved but seems very reluctant to have him stay with her, and she has not followed through on obtaining power of attorney. I wonder if he might have "depression with reversible dementia syndrome"; these patients typically have more psychic and somatic anxiety symptoms than other dementia patients, and there is potential for significant cognitive improvement with treatment of depression [18]. His psychiatrist agrees that his cognitive function might improve with antidepressant treatment, but this could take 4–6 weeks or more. Our plan at this point is to transfer him to a nursing home with a dementia care unit and reevaluate his capacity next month.

3. Ms. Lee is a 68-year-old woman with gallstone pancreatitis complicated by a large pseudocyst that has not responded to conservative treatment. Despite 2 weeks of bowel rest and TPN, she continues to have intractable nausea, vomiting, and epigastric pain, and the pseudocyst has increased in size to 5×8 cm on CT. Optimal treatment for symptomatic pseudocysts depends on the location and size of the pseudocyst, its distance from the stomach or duodenum, and whether or not it communicates with the pancreatic duct. Internal drainage with endoscopic cystogastrostomy, cysto-duodenostomy, or transpapillary drainage is now the preferred initial approach for most symptomatic pseudocysts [19]. Endoscopic ultrasound (EUS) is the method of choice for the evaluation of pancreatic pseudocysts because it can accurately measure the distance between the GI tract lumen and the pseudocyst and also identify varices or peri-pancreatic collaterals that might increase risk for bleeding

complications [20]. In Ms. Lee's case, the pseudocyst is in the body of the pancreas and was found by EUS to be <1 cm from the gastric lumen, so we have opted for endoscopic cystogastrostomy. The clinical success rate for this procedure is nearly 90%; possible complications include bleeding, perforation, sepsis, and pancreatic fistula.

The Evidence-Infused Assessment

Note that every one of these assessments is made better with a focused literature search to answer a specific question. What is the differential diagnosis for a right-sided, transudative pleural effusion? What are the symptoms of baclofen withdrawal? What is clinical futility? It's very important for students to understand that we do not have textbook chapters or randomized controlled trials to answer all of the diagnostic and treatment questions that arise on the wards and in the clinic. We must use the best available evidence. Case reports, case series, review articles, guidelines, case-control and cohort studies, and articles on mechanisms of disease can be used to argue for a diagnosis and devise a treatment plan. With the era of personalized medicine upon us, our conceptions of the value of evidence are becoming more fluid. Pertinence is what really counts; pedantic pronouncements about the "evidence hierarchy" are becoming less relevant when it comes to caring for the individual patient. "Hierarchies are a poor basis for the application of evidence in clinical practice," writes Christopher Blunt. Hierarchies provide estimates of differential average treatment effects, but "information about the distribution of effects and the causes and predictors of effect heterogeneity" is most important for clinicians and their patients [21]. This information can come from many sources. *The key is to find the best evidence, in whatever form, that fits the case.* Search broadly; if you limit yourself to randomized controlled trials and meta-analyses, you might not find the decisive evidence that could clinch the diagnosis or optimize treatment.

Let us know what you're thinking, then, but show us the evidence. Your assessment is a thesis: it must be argued for and defended. Prepare your argument in advance. Support it with a focused and pertinent literature search. Cite the evidence as part of your oral presentation. Use your fresh knowledge of basic science to create a hypothesis when there is an unexplained or unexpected event. Infuse your assessment with the best and most specific evidence you can find.

References

1. Strohl M, Packer C. When asthma is not asthma. JGIM Clinical Images 2015 January 14. http://www.sgim.org/web-only/clinical-images/when-asthma-is-not-asthma. Accessed 18 Aug 2018.
2. Zias N, Chroneou A, Tabba MK, Gonzalez AV, Gray AW, Lamb CR, et al. Post tracheostomy and post intubation tracheal stenosis: report of 31 cases and review of the literature. BMC Pulm Med. 2008;8:18.
3. Porcel JM, Light RW. Diagnostic approach to pleural effusion in adults. Am Fam Physician. 2006;73(7):1211–20.
4. Porcel JM. Pleural effusions from congestive heart failure. Semin Respir Crit Care Med. 2010;31(6):689–97.
5. Sureka B, Bansal K, Patidar Y, Kumar S, Arora A. Thoracic perspective revisited in chronic liver disease. Gastroenterol Rep (Oxf). 2015;3(3):194–200.
6. Badillo R, Rockey DC. Hepatic hydrothorax: clinical features, management, and outcomes in 77 patients and review of the literature. Medicine (Baltimore). 2014;93(3):135–42.
7. Eid AA, Keddissi JI, Kinasewitz GT. Hypoalbuminemia as a cause of pleural effusions. Chest. 1999;115(4):1066–9.
8. Foschi FG, Piscaglia F, Pompili M, Corbelli C, Marano G, Righini R, et al. Real-time contrast-enhanced ultrasound – a new simple tool for detection of peritoneal-pleural communications in hepatic hydrothorax. Ultraschall Med. 2008;29(5):538–42.
9. Hanna EB. Syncope: etiology and diagnostic approach. Cleve Clin J Med. 2014;81(12):755–66.
10. Park JJ, Park S, Choi D. Microvascular angina: angina that predominantly affects women. Korean J Intern Med. 2015;30(2):140–7.

11. Braun MM, Barstow CH, Pyzocha NJ. Diagnosis and management of sodium disorders: hyponatremia and hypernatremia. Am Fam Physician. 2015;91(5):299–307.
12. Wells PS, Anderson DR, Rodger M, Forgie M, Kearon C, Dreyer J, et al. Evaluation of D-dimer in the diagnosis of suspected deep-vein thrombosis. N Engl J Med. 2003;349(13):1227–35.
13. Helliwell T, Hider SL. Diagnosis and management of polymyalgia rheumatica. Br J Gen Pract. 2012;62(598):275–6.
14. Leo RJ, Baer D. Delirium associated with baclofen withdrawal: a review of common presentations and management strategies. Psychosomatics. 2005;46(6):503–7.
15. D'Aleo G, Cammaroto S, Rifici C, Marra G, Sessa E, Bramanti P, et al. Hallucinations after abrupt withdrawal of oral and intrathecal baclofen. Funct Neurol. 2007;22(2):81–8.
16. Kraut JA, Kurtz I. Toxic alcohol ingestions: clinical features, diagnosis, and management. Clin J Am Soc Nephrol. 2008;3(1):208–25.
17. Kasman DL. When is medical treatment futile? A guide for students, residents, and physicians. J Gen Intern Med. 2004;19(10):1053–6.
18. Morimoto SS, Kanellopoulos D, Manning KJ, Alexopoulos GS. Diagnosis and treatment of depression and cognitive impairment in late-life. Ann N Y Acad Sci. 2015;1345(1):36–46.
19. Pan G, Wan MH, Xie K, Li W, Hu WM, Liu XB, et al. Classification and management of pancreatic pseudocysts. Medicine (Baltimore). 2015;94(24):e960.
20. Saftoiu A, Vilmann A, Vilmann P. Endoscopic ultrasound-guided drainage of pancreatic pseudocysts. Endosc Ultrasound. 2015;4(4):319–23.
21. Blunt CJ. Hierarchies of evidence in evidence-based medicine. Doctoral thesis. London: London School of Economics; 2015.
22. Lanza GA, Buffon A, Sestito A, Natale L, Sgueglia GA, Galiuto L, et al. Relation between stress-induced myocardial perfusion defects on cardiovascular magnetic resonance and coronary microvascular dysfunction in patients with cardiac syndrome X. J Am Coll Cardiol. 2008;51(4):466–72.

Chapter 8
Approaches to Differential Diagnosis

In describing their own methods of inquiry, clinicians speak of "experience, trial and error, intuition, and muddling through." In actuality, this process involves pattern recognition skills too complex to be duplicated by a computer. [1]

James D. Sapira

Students must be taught to acquire a capacity for the "sustained muddleheadedness" and the tolerance for ambiguity…so essential when difficult unexplained findings are dealt with. A diagnosis is a step forward only when it can be sustained by the evidence at hand. [2]

Lawrence Weed

Active Diagnosis: Hypothesis Testing in Real Time

New medical students typically think that the diagnostic process consists of seeing and examining a patient, collecting a treasure trove of miscellaneous clinical data, and then retreating to a quiet room to make sense of the findings. This method – passive data collection followed by diagnostic reflection – is an inefficient way to put together a differential diagnosis. For one thing, the student (who is working through the differential after the fact) will keep remembering questions that were not asked or physical exam findings that need to be rechecked. This can make for multiple trips back to the bedside, disturbing the peace of the increasingly impatient patient, who is trying to get some sleep. Another problem with this approach is that, with so many shiny and interesting objects in the treasure chest, it can be very hard to decide which ones to keep and which to throw away.

The solution to this problem, which most students figure out eventually, is to take an *active* approach with the history and physical exam. This means using questions and exam findings to test a series of diagnostic hypotheses *in real time* as you take the history and perform the physical. In the case of a patient presenting with abdominal pain, this means asking a series of specific questions to test several diagnostic possibilities:

1. *Biliary colic*: Where do you feel the pain? Does it build up gradually, become very intense, and then ease up gradually? Does it wake you up at night? Did you have any nausea or vomiting? What did you have for supper on the night it woke you up? Does the pain radiate to your right shoulder blade area? Did you notice any yellowness in your eyes or skin? Any dark urine or light-colored stool? Have you had pains like this in the past? Have you ever been told that you have gallstones?

2. *Peptic ulcer disease*: Does the pain get better or worse with eating? Did you try antacids? How long after eating does the pain start up again? Does it wake you up at night? What can you do to relieve the pain? Is there any black stool or blood in the stool? Are you taking aspirin or NSAID pain medicines, such as ibuprofen or naproxen? Have you ever been told that you have an ulcer or had an upper GI endoscopy?

3. *Acute pancreatitis*: Is the pain constant or intermittent? Does it radiate to the middle of your back? Is it better when you sit up? Do you have nausea or vomiting? Do you drink alcohol? How much alcohol have you been drinking lately? Have you ever had gallstones? Any new medications? Any similar pain episodes in the past?

4. *Nephrolithiasis*: Do you feel the pain in your back or flank? Does it radiate to the groin? Does it build up gradually, become very intense, and then ease up gradually? Any nausea or vomiting? Any blood in the urine? Have you passed any stones or particles in the urine?

This blending of data collection and analysis requires a certain mental dexterity at first, until the process becomes automatic through repetition and experience. Whether the chief complaint is chest pain, acute onset of confusion, or a swollen left elbow with fever, active diagnosis means following your line of questioning, wherever it leads. The goal should be to emerge from the patient's room with a provisional diagnosis as well as a thorough history and physical.

Diagnostic Theories, Principles, and Caveats

Medical students should have a basic understanding of the various theories and principles of diagnosis, as well as the biases and errors that may frustrate their diagnostic efforts. Self-reflection is a very important part of the learning process, and mistakes can be hard to pinpoint if there is no theoretical framework to fall back on. Diagnosis is an incredibly complex process. Rules and methods can be helpful, but they do not fully comprehend or explain the multi-level processing that occurs in the mind of an experienced physician. Think of the following concepts as guideposts to help you find your own way as a diagnostician.

Occam's Razor

The English philosopher William of Occam (c.1287–1347) had among his many accomplishments a theory of efficient reasoning, which has come to be known as Occam's Razor. His aphorism, *Pluralitas non est ponenda sine necessitate* (plurality must not be posited without necessity), is often applied to medical diagnosis. In other words, "among competing hypotheses, the simplest explanation is the best," or "try to fit as many symptoms as possible under the umbrella of a single disease." This diagnostic parsimony can lead to elegant, efficient, and cost-effective medical care. I recently took care of a patient with a bioprosthetic aortic valve who presented with high fever and severe back pain. His examination was significant for a 3/6 systolic ejection murmur at the left sternal border, thoracic spinous tenderness, and splinter hemorrhages in several fingernails. MRI revealed vertebral osteomyelitis and discitis at multiple levels in the thoracic spine, and CT of the abdomen showed splenic and renal infarcts. Blood cultures grew *Strep sanguinis* and *Staph hominis*. Most experienced physicians would immediately recognize that all of these hematogenous infections and infarcts could result from one disease: prosthetic valve endocarditis. Transesophageal echocardiography confirmed the diagnosis with findings of valvular vegetations and a paravalvular abscess. (See below for examples of how to apply Occam's diagnostic parsimony to a variety of cases using "The Law of Sigma" and "The Key Findings Approach.")

Hickam's Dictum

As it turns out, adherence to Occam's Razor is an aspirational goal that is sometimes unattainable in actual medical practice. Our patients have an inconvenient habit of showing up with more than one disease at a time, or with many unrelated symptoms. For example, a typical patient might complain of chronic bilateral ankle swelling, right lower ribcage pain, dysuria, vertigo, a tickling cough, a lump on the left calf, and a sore spot under the right scapula. What is the unifying diagnosis? One of my most complicated patients (a practical joker) once pulled a thick scroll of paper out of his pocket and told me it was a list of his symptoms for the visit. As I groaned inwardly, he suddenly dropped the scroll, and it unrolled across the room, revealing about 15 ft of blank paper. After I recovered myself, we had a great laugh together. As I reflected on the incident later, it occurred to me that the scroll embodies the idea that multiple diseases and proliferating symptoms are the rule rather than the exception.

Thus the counterpoint to Occam's Razor, which is known as Hickam's Dictum: "A man can have as many diseases as he damn well pleases." Dr. John Hickam was chief of medicine at Indiana University from 1958 to 1970, and his now-famous dictum was an expression of his frustration with the limitations of Occam's Razor in dealing with the complexities of diagnosis in the real world. By all means try the Occamite method first when you are confronted with a diagnostic challenge. When it all fits together, nothing could be more satisfying. But don't force it. Trying to fit square pegs into round holes for the sake of parsimony can lead to serious diagnostic errors.

The Law of Sigma

This is a corollary of Occam's Razor. If a patient who is known to have Disease A presents with new symptoms, it is best to consider rare or unusual manifestations of Disease A before positing a completely new diagnosis, Disease B [1]. In Fig. 8.1, the crest of each sine wave represents the common manifestations of Disease A and Disease B. The downsloping sides of the waves represent the rare or unusual manifestations of each disease.

Consider the following scenarios in which applying the Law of Sigma (1) leads directly to the diagnosis and (2) lowers the cost of the diagnostic work-up. (All cost estimates for diagnostic tests and are from healthcarebluebook.com.)

Disease A   Disease B

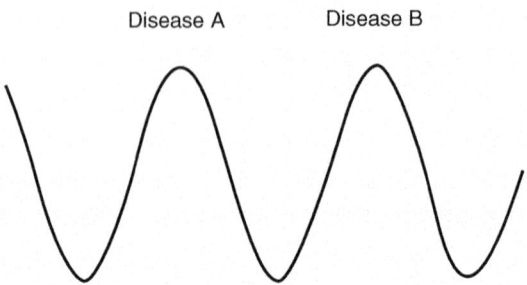

FIGURE 8.1 The Law of Sigma

Case 1

A 35-year-old man with a seizure disorder presents with 1 day of:

- Nystagmus
- Ataxic gait
- Orthostatic hypotension

What is your diagnosis?

If we bypass the seizure disorder and consider the presenting symptoms as a totally new diagnosis, we would probably want an MRI of the brain ($969) to rule out a brainstem or cerebellar stroke. If we follow the Law of Sigma and begin by considering more unusual manifestations of the patient's know seizure disorder (including treatment), it might eventually occur to us that the patient has classic symptoms of phenytoin toxicity. An elevated phenytoin level ($34) would clinch the diagnosis.

Case 2

A 55-year-old woman with metastatic breast cancer presents with:

- Lethargy without focal neurologic findings
- Diffuse abdominal pain
- Polyuria

What is your diagnosis?

If we bypass the known metastatic breast cancer and posit a new diagnosis, we would probably order a slew of diagnostic tests, including a non-contrast head CT ($303) and an abdominal CT with and without contrast ($559). But by starting with the metastatic breast cancer and considering its possible metabolic complications, we would arrive at the diagnosis of hypercalcemia, which explains all of her symptoms and could be confirmed with a simple serum calcium ($13).

Case 3

An 80-year-old man with HTN, CAD, and hypothyroidism presents with:

- Progressive leg edema
- Shortness of breath
- Enlarged heart on chest x-ray
- Moderate pericardial effusion on echocardiogram

What is the cause of this patient's pericardial effusion?

The differential diagnosis for pericardial effusion includes pericarditis, malignancy, viral infections, autoimmune diseases, tuberculosis, nephrotic syndrome, and heart failure. If we bypass the patient's known medical conditions, the differential remains broad, and a diagnostic pericardiocentesis ($2876) would probably be required. However, myxedema is also a rare cause of pericardial effusion, and further investigation revealed that this patient had stopped taking his levothyroxine when the prescription ran out 6 months before. His TSH ($54) was 70 mIU/L, consistent with profound hypothyroidism. The effusion gradually resolved with resumption of levothyroxine treatment.

Obviously, the Law of Sigma (like Occam's Razor) cannot be applied in all cases. New symptoms are often brought on by new diseases. However, a good diagnostician carefully considers the whole spectrum of a known diagnosis before moving on to a new one.

Post Hoc Ergo Propter Hoc

To understand the post hoc ergo propter hoc fallacy, consider this case from my own clinical practice. A 62-year-old man developed a severe, burning pain that radiated from his right shoulder down to the wrist. He went immediately to his local drugstore and bought a tube of aspirin cream, which he applied liberally to the painful area. A short time later, he broke out in a painful blistering rash down the arm, where he had just applied the cream. He went to the emergency room where a physician heard the story, looked at the blistering rash, and diagnosed him with an allergic reaction to the aspirin cream. The patient took diphenhydramine as prescribed, but the pain continued to worsen even as the rash faded. A month later he came to my office, sleeping poorly and suffering agonizing pain in his arm. It was obvious from his description of his burning pain and the dermatomal distribution of the rash that my patient had shingles. So why had the ER physician missed such a simple diagnosis? It was the temporal association between the aspirin cream and the rash. Post hoc ergo propter hoc means "if A follows B, A was caused by B," or "a temporal association implies causation." Pain frequently precedes the rash in herpes zoster [3], and my patient's presentation was typical for shingles. The ER physician was certainly aware of the natural history of shingles and had probably diagnosed it many times, but the timing of the aspirin cream skewed the picture. Similarly, when a patient presents with fever that resolves after antibiotic treatment, don't assume that the antibiotic "cured" the fever, especially if all of the patient's cultures are negative.

Heuristics

Medical heuristics have been described as "the silent adjudicators of clinical practice" [4]. Heuristics are cognitive shortcuts that allow physicians to make quick diagnostic and treatment decisions in their daily practices. In essence, heuristics are simple, efficient rules of thumb based on experience and common sense, a form of "fast and frugal" decision-making in settings where there is limited information and limited time. The rapid pattern recognition used so impressively by master diagnosticians is probably the highest form of heuristic reasoning. Interestingly, heuristics often outperform complex diagnostic algorithms and prediction tools when it comes to diagnostic accuracy. "One reason for the surprising performance of heuristics," writes Julian Marewski, "is that they ignore information. This makes them quicker to execute, easier to understand, and easier to communicate" [5]. For example, a commonly used heuristic for assessment of chest pain – Is it substernal? Is it exertional? Is it relieved with nitroglycerin? – is a powerful predictor of angina pectoris even in the absence of other information, such as cardiovascular disease risk scores. Another heuristic, "In pneumonia, when fever and leukocytosis persist after more than 48 hours of appropriate antibiotic treatment, suspect an empyema," helps physicians to decide when repeat imaging should be done in cases of complicated pneumonia.

It should be noted that heuristic reasoning is mostly out of reach for medical students. Rapid pattern recognition requires extensive experience. Medical students who think they can make an instant diagnosis are in for a rude awakening. Metacognition (thinking about thinking) is the opposite of heuristic reasoning; it is the awareness and understanding of one's own thought processes. Medical students practice metacognition as they analyze, test, and refute various diagnostic possibilities. Students can also learn to use metacognition to identify the pitfalls and biases that lead to misdiagnosis.

Heuristic Failures and Diagnostic Biases

The conclusions we draw from heuristics are often correct, but unfortunately they are also subject to a variety of biases (Table 8.1) that may lead to diagnostic errors. The best defense against these errors is a willingness to analyze one's

TABLE 8.1   Heuristic failures

Heuristic	Description
Anchoring bias	Tendency to lock on to the early features of a presentation and not adjust initial impression in light of later information
Confirmation bias	The tendency to seek confirming evidence to support a diagnosis rather than look for elements that would refute the hypothesis
Availability bias	Disposition to judge a diagnosis as more likely if you have seen it more recently or if it comes more easily to mind
Diagnosis momentum	The tendency for a diagnosis to become "stickier" with repetition
Framing effect	The perceived likelihood of a diagnosis is influenced by the way it is presented
Sunk-cost bias	Unwillingness to abandon a diagnosis in which considerable effort has been expended
Premature closure	The tendency to accept a decision before it is completely verified, also called satisfied search phenomenon
Visceral bias	Emotional arousal leads to poor decision making. The clinician may overweight the diagnosis that he or she wants to be true
Triage cueing	The initial selection of location or specialist has disproportionate influence on subsequent care
Multiple-alternatives bias	The attempt to simplify a list of multiple potential possibilities to a less-complex list by ignoring some options

Reprinted with permission from Cumbler and Trosterman [6]

own reasoning and consider the cognitive traps of quick decision-making. As Cumbler and Trosterman state in *The Psychology of Error*, "a moment spent to reflect on how you came to a diagnosis may be time well spent" [6].

Heuristic failures are common. Consider two cases presented by my third-year medicine clerkship students. The first was a man with recently diagnosed lung cancer and a history of heart failure who presented with shortness of breath and bilateral pleural effusions. Since bilateral pleural effusions are generally transudates, the attending decided to forego a diagnostic tap and treat the patient for heart failure with furosemide. The patient returned a few days later with shortness of breath and worsening effusions, and thoracentesis revealed an exudate with cytology positive for adenocarcinoma. This is an example of premature closure, where a diagnosis was made before it was completely verified. In the other case, a man was hospitalized with pneumonia and found to have pancytopenia and borderline neutropenia. A hematologist was consulted, who attributed the pancytopenia to the patient's infection. The patient was discharged on antibiotics but continued to do poorly. He was readmitted 3 weeks later with severe neutropenia, fever, and sepsis and was subsequently diagnosed with acute myelogenous leukemia (AML). While it is true that some viral infections and overwhelming bacterial infections can cause pancytopenia, the possibility of a hematologic malignancy or other bone marrow disorders was ignored. This led to a catastrophic delay in the diagnosis of AML. Anchoring bias and the framing effect both contributed to this unfortunate outcome.

Cognitive forcing strategies can help to guard against heuristic failures. One strategy is to make deliberate use of the differential diagnosis in every case (see below), even when the first impression seems to suggest a clear and obvious diagnosis. A second strategy is to include diagnostic uncertainty as part of the checkout at all transitions of care, which can help to prevent the propagation of diagnostic bias and error from one physician to another [6].

The Key Findings Approach to Differential Diagnosis

The key findings approach to differential diagnosis (see also Chaps. 2, 5, and 7) works well for medical students. It is a simple, stepwise process that leads to a prioritized differential diagnosis and a rational testing strategy. Experienced diagnosticians often fall back on this approach in very complicated cases where heuristics fail and the patterns are hard to recognize.

Step 1 is to identify the key findings from the history, physical exam, lab and imaging results, and initial response to treatment. For example, consider a patient who presents with the following key findings:

- Pleuritic chest pain
- Shortness of breath
- Tachycardia
- Tachypnea
- Positive D-dimer

Step 2 is to identify the leading finding, which will be used to develop a differential diagnosis. The leading finding is *not* the most dramatic, unusual, or life-threatening sign or symptom; it is the one with the shortest list of possible causes. This limits the differential diagnosis and makes for a more manageable and efficient work-up.

- Pleuritic chest pain: limited possibilities – pleurisy, chest wall pain, pneumonia, and pulmonary embolism; *best choice for the leading finding*
- Shortness of breath: many possible causes
- Tachycardia: many possible causes
- Tachypnea: many possible causes
- Positive D-dimer: non-specific test, many possible causes; more helpful diagnostically if negative

There are hundreds of possible causes of dyspnea, tachycardia, and tachypnea, but pleuritic chest pain gives us a manageable list of possibilities.

Consider another case with the following key findings:

- History of depression
- Shortness of breath
- Respiratory alkalosis
- Anion gap metabolic acidosis
- Progression to pulmonary edema

A patient with a history of depression develops shortness of breath, acid-base disorders, and progresses to pulmonary edema. The story strongly suggests a toxic ingestion. Which is the leading finding?

- History of depression: might be important, but is not the leading finding
- Shortness of breath: many possible causes
- Respiratory alkalosis: many possible causes, including pulmonary embolism, pneumonia, sepsis, asthma, cirrhosis, toxic ingestions (salicylate), hypoxemia, acute anxiety, pneumothorax, meningitis, encephalitis, brain tumor
- Anion gap metabolic acidosis: the four main causes are toxic ingestions (methanol, ethylene glycol, and salicylate are most common), lactic acidosis, ketoacidosis, and renal failure; *best choice for the leading finding*
- Pulmonary edema: many possible causes, including heart failure, ARDS, viral infections, high altitude, smoke inhalation, neurogenic, viral infections, pulmonary embolism, and numerous drugs and toxins

Again, the short list of possibilities for an anion gap acidosis makes it a good starting point for the differential diagnosis.

Step 3. Create a broad differential diagnosis based on the leading finding. For medical students, this usually requires a source with differential diagnosis lists, either online

(UpToDate, Diagnosaurus) or one of the various pocket differential diagnosis handbooks. A broad differential is important to rule out unusual diseases and account for all possibilities. For instance, rare causes of pleuritic chest pain can include epipericardial fat necrosis [7], familial Mediterranean fever [8], and nitrofurantoin pulmonary toxicity [9], among others. Other toxic ingestions that can cause an anion gap metabolic acidosis include overdoses of metformin [10] and isoniazid [11].

Step 4. Once the broad differential diagnosis is established, read about the possibilities and discuss them with more experienced clinicians, to see which can be discarded and which might fit. This is the process of narrowing the differential and establishing a working diagnosis. In the case of the patient with pleuritic chest pain, the shortness of breath, tachypnea, tachycardia, and + D-dimer all point to a working diagnosis of pulmonary embolism. For the patient with an anion gap metabolic acidosis and possible drug ingestion, further reading reveals that respiratory alkalosis followed by anion gap metabolic acidosis is the classic pattern for salicylate toxicity and that some patients will progress to pulmonary edema. Salicylate toxicity becomes the working diagnosis.

Step 5. Develop a testing strategy to confirm the working diagnosis or to decide among competing diagnoses. Chest CT is the gold standard for diagnosing pulmonary embolism, and a high salicylate level would confirm the aspirin overdose. For a middle-aged man with no prior history of gout presenting with a hot, swollen knee, the differential would include gout, pseudogout, inflammatory arthritis, and septic joint. A knee aspiration for crystals, cell counts, gram stain, and culture would be the ideal diagnostic test. For a patient with fever, lymphadenopathy, a palmar rash, and a working diagnosis of secondary syphilis, an RPR would be the test of choice. RPR is 100% sensitive for secondary syphilis, so a negative result would rule out the diagnosis. Specificity is 85–99%, so a highly specific treponemal test such as the FTA-ABS would be required to confirm the diagnosis after a positive RPR. A clear understanding of test characteristics and Bayesian reasoning is essential at this stage. Remember that a differential diagnosis without a testing strategy is a job only partially done. The testing strategy requires much thought, reading, and discussion. To save time, review diagnostic criteria and approaches to testing at the same time you read about each possibility in the differential diagnosis.

Using the Key Findings Approach in a Complex Case

The patient is a 48-year-old man who presented with a 4-day history of fevers and chills as well as pain in the fourth and fifth MCP joints in the right hand. Two to three days before admission, he had also noted "bumps" developing on his face, neck, back, and legs. His ROS was negative for dysuria, diarrhea, visual changes, or penile discharge. However, he did recall having a sore throat 2 weeks prior to the onset of other symptoms.

His past medical history was significant for hypertension. He was taking no medications. He denied alcohol, tobacco, or illicit drug use.

On physical exam, he was a thin black man in moderate distress. He was febrile to 102.4° with BP 100/64, HR 110, and RR 22. Multiple 1–2 cm salmon-colored nodules were noted on his neck, back, and legs. There was swelling, erythema, and tenderness involving the fourth and fifth MCP joints of the right hand. He had cervical, axillary, epitrochlear, and inguinal lymphadenopathy. No cardiac murmurs were appreciated. Lung, abdominal, and GU exams were unremarkable, and there was no pharyngeal erythema or exudate.

Labs were significant for WBC 12,300, AST 201, ALT 207, LDH 290, alkaline phosphatase 204, and ESR 103. Urinalysis was unremarkable. CXR and ECG were normal. Multiple blood cultures were negative.

During his hospital stay, the patient developed a right knee effusion. Aspiration revealed 2400 WBC/cmm with negative crystal examination, gram stain, and culture. He also developed left eye pain and redness; ophthalmologic examination showed episcleritis. An echocardiogram was performed and interpreted as normal. Liver biopsy was normal. Biopsy of a skin nodule showed erythema nodosum.

The patient was started on high-dose aspirin with resolution of his fever and skin nodules and improvement in his joint symptoms. A diagnostic test was performed in the hospital and repeated 3 weeks later on an outpatient basis.

(Diagnosic test: the antistreptolysin-O (ASO) titer was 198 on admission (normal 0–200). Two weeks later, the ASO titer was 352).

This is an actual case from my time attending on the VA wards many years ago. I vividly recall working through the differential diagnosis and constructing a table with the key findings and diagnostic possibilities to help organize my thinking. My list of key findings:

- Migratory polyarthritis
- Fever
- Lymphadenopathy
- Subcutaneous nodules
- Erythema nodosum
- Abnormal liver function tests
- Episcleritis
- Resolution with aspirin

Since there are a limited number of diseases that cause migratory polyarthritis, it is a good choice to be the leading finding in this case. Although migratory polyarthritis is classically seen in rheumatic fever, it can occur in several other inflammatory, infectious, and allergic diseases, including adult Still's disease, serum sickness, sarcoidosis, Sweet's syndrome, and a few others. In Table 8.2, the key findings are listed in the left-hand column, and the differential diagnosis for migratory

TABLE 8.2 Diagnostic table for a complex case of migratory polyarthritis with fever

	Rheumatic fever	Serum sickness	Adult still's	IBD	Sarcoid	Hep B	Sweet's syndrome	SLE	Gonococcal arthritis
Migratory polyarthritis	+ (2/3)	+	+ (large joints)	+ (migratory)	+/– (can be migratory)	(or arthralgias)	+	+ (migratory)	+ (migratory)
Fever	+	+	+ (high)	+	+ (10–15%)	+	+	+	+
Lymphadenopathy	–	+/–	+	–	+ (25%)	–	+	+	–
SC nodules	+	–	+/–	–	+ (25%)	–	–	–	–
Erythema nodosum	+/–	–	–	+	+	+	+/–	–	–
Abnl LFT	–	–	+ (73%)	+/–	+	+	–	–	–
Episcleritis	–	–	+ (uveitis)	+	+ (uveitis)	?	–	+	–
Resolution with ASA	+	–	+ (25%)	–	–	–	–	–	–
Comments:	*For:* High ASO titer Prior sore throat *Against:* Age Small joints involved Atypical distribution of SC nodules Abnl LFT Erythema nodosum LAN and eye involvement	*For:* Polyathritis and fever *Against:* Urticarial rash usual No recent PCN/ cephalosporin Many red herrings	*For:* 92% w/ sore throat Triad of fever, rash, arthritis *Against:* Predominantly female, peak age 16–35 Asymmetric arthritis unusual Not typical Still's rash	*Against:* No GI symptoms	*For:* Few red herrings *Against:* 90% have abnormal CXR 80% have + skin or liver biopsy Normal ACE and Ca levels Fulminant onset	*Against:* Purpuric skin lesions usual Neg. serology	*Against:* No underlying lympho-proliferative disease Rash typically dermal infiltrate	*Against:* Neg. ANA Insufficient clinical criteria	*Against:* Neg. sexual history Many red herrings

polyarthritis is given across the top row. The diagnostician's next task is to fill in the rest of the table, in order to see how many of the key findings fit with each diagnosis. This usually requires a concentrated bout of reading and discussion, especially when there is no obvious working diagnosis. In this case, three main possibilities emerge: rheumatic fever, adult Still's disease, and sarcoidosis. The "comments" at the bottom of the table give the arguments for and against each of these diagnoses. In the end, the patient was treated for rheumatic fever with penicillin prophylaxis, although adult Still's and sarcoidosis could not be ruled out. This case illustrates the probabilistic nature of diagnosis; physicians must learn to accept that absolute certainty is rare and that ranking diagnostic probabilities and making treatment decisions are the day-to-day work of all doctors who see patients.

References

1. Sapira JD. The art & science of bedside diagnosis. Baltimore: Urban and Schwarzenberg; 1990.
2. Weed LL. Medical records that guide and teach. N Engl J Med. 1968;278(11):593–600.
3. Wood M. Understanding pain in herpes zoster: an essential for optimizing treatment. J Infect Dis. 2002;186(Suppl 1):S78–82.
4. McDonald CJ. Medical heuristics: the silent adjudicators of clinical practice. Ann Intern Med. 1996;124(1 Pt 1):56–62.
5. Marewski JN. Heuristic decision making in medicine. Dialogues Clin Neurosci. 2012;14(1):77–89.
6. Cumbler E, Trosterman A. The Psychology of Error. The Hospitalist. 2007;11(11):34–35.
7. Runge T, Greganti MA. Epipericardial fat necrosis – a rare cause of pleuritic chest pain: case report and review of the literature. Arch Med Sci. 2011;7(2):337–41.
8. Ozkaya S, Butun SE, Findik S, Atici A, Dirican A. A very rare cause of pleuritic chest pain: bilateral pleuritis as a first sign of familial Mediterranean fever. Case Rep Pulmonol. 2013;2013:315751.
9. Caponi B. An unusual cause of pleuritic chest pain. [Abstract]. J Hosp Med. 2013;8(suppl 2).

10. Timbrell S, Wilbourn G, Harper J, Liddle A. Lactic acidosis secondary to metformin overdose: a case report. J Med Case Rep. 2012;6:230.
11. Alvarez FG, Guntupalli KK. Isoniazid overdose: four case reports and review of the literature. Intensive Care Med. 1995;21(8):641–4.

Chapter 9
Searching and Citing the Literature

Using the Literature Search to Optimize Patient Care

As a medical student, one of the most important ways you can contribute to your patient's care is to perform a thorough literature search. Interns and residents are very busy admitting and caring for large numbers of patients, and their care decisions tend to be driven by guidelines, protocols, and the opinions of their attending physicians. Searching the literature takes time, and extra time is often lacking for physicians in training. Medical students, on the other hand, have the luxury of time and are expected to dig deeper and take a more scholarly approach to their work. Sometimes that extra digging can result in better outcomes for patients.

In Chap. 7, I presented several hypothetical examples of student assessments where a focused literature search helped to narrow the differential diagnosis and answer the specific questions raised by the case. Here are a few actual cases from my own experience as an attending on the VA wards, where my students' literature searches led directly to better patient care:

1. A 64-year-old man was admitted with an asthma exacerbation. He had a history of severe asthma with almost monthly hospitalizations over the past year, including two ICU admissions where he had been intubated for several days.

© Springer Nature Switzerland AG 2019
C. D. Packer, *Presenting Your Case*,
https://doi.org/10.1007/978-3-030-13792-2_9

The medical student did a careful chart review and found that he had had eosinophilia with every admission, as well as migratory pulmonary infiltrates with consistently negative sputum and blood cultures (there were no comments on the eosinophilia in the previous hospital notes). She performed a literature search and came up with a working diagnosis of Churg-Strauss vasculitis [1]. She discussed her findings with the team and consulted a rheumatologist, who agreed with the diagnosis. Lung biopsy revealed eosinophilic vasculitis, and the patient was started on immunosuppressive treatment in addition to corticosteroids. There were no further hospital admissions for asthma.

2. A 53-year-old man with metastatic bladder cancer was admitted for severe chemotherapy-induced diarrhea (CID). He had recently been discharged after a 3-week hospitalization for intractable CID complicated by acute renal failure despite treatment with aggressive IV hydration and a high-dose loperamide regimen. As we braced ourselves for another long and difficult hospitalization, the medical student who admitted him searched the literature and found a small prospective trial of subcutaneous octreotide for patients with loperamide-refractory CID. In the trial, 94% of the patients had complete resolution of their diarrhea within 24–72 h [2]. Subcutaneous octreotide is very expensive, and it was a non-formulary drug at that time. The student convinced us to try the octreotide, arguing that the cost would be offset by a greatly shortened hospitalization; she then worked with a pharmacist to get the non-formulary drug approval. The octreotide worked like a charm, and the patient was discharged from the hospital after 24 hours of treatment.

3. An 82-year-old man presented with weight loss and failure to thrive. In the course of his work-up, he was found to have a hard, nodular prostate and a PSA of 200 ng/mL. His metastatic work-up revealed multiple lung nodules that were suspicious for metastases, but no bone or liver lesions. I had never heard of prostate cancer metastatic only to the lungs and suspected a second malignancy. Plans were made for a diagnostic bronchoscopy, but the medical student

who was caring for him searched the literature and found several case reports of prostate cancer metastatic only to the lungs, with complete regression of the lung metastases after hormonal treatment [3]. Armed with this new information, we cancelled the bronchoscopy and consulted with an oncologist, who reviewed the case and agreed with the plan to start antiandrogen therapy. The student's literature search had expedited the patient's cancer treatment and prevented an unnecessary procedure [4].

In each of these instances, the medical student identified the key question raised by the case:

- Why does this patient with intractable asthma have persistent eosinophilia?
- Is there an alternative treatment for chemotherapy-induced diarrhea that is refractory to loperamide?
- Does prostate cancer sometimes metastasize only to the lungs?

Each student then researched the question, presented the findings to the team, and made a convincing argument for a change of course that ultimately benefitted the patient. For a medical student, this is clearly honors-level work. At a certain point, this goes beyond a well-applied literature search and becomes pure patient advocacy. I recall that the student who cared for the CID patient was very persistent and even passionate about trying the octreotide; she overcame both the inertia of our established treatment plan and our skepticism due to the limited evidence and high cost of treatment. She made certain that her patient got the best possible care. She (and the others) showed that third-year medical students can make a difference for their patients.

How to Search the Literature

You have diagnosed a patient in the clinic with primary hyperaldosteronism and will need to start him on an aldosterone antagonist. The question is whether to start him on spironolactone or eplerenone. You know that spironolactone is less expensive, but it can cause gynecomastia. Which drug is more likely to control the patient's hypertension?

There are many ways to search the literature. A Google web search using the phrase "spironolactone versus eplerenone for primary hyperaldosteronism" produces about 28,700 results, but (happily) the 3 most relevant randomized clinical trials appear on the first web page. One trial [5] showed significantly better blood pressure control with spironolactone; the other two [6, 7] concluded that both drugs were equally effective. The problem with web searches is the huge denominator: 3 out of 27,800 is a search with distressingly poor specificity. The handful of significant studies can easily be lost in a sea of marginally relevant articles, web pages, news reports, and so forth, especially if they don't happen to appear in the first page or two. Nevertheless, a focused web search can be a good starting point. "For many clinical scenarios," writes Mohammad Al-Ubaydli, "Google and other search engines can provide, quickly enough, an answer that is good enough [8]."

A better option for searching the literature for answers to specific clinical questions is the PubMed MeSH (Medical Subject Heading) search. PubMed is a service of the US National Library of Medicine that provides free online access to the MEDLINE database of indexed citations and abstracts to medical, nursing, dental, veterinary, health care, and pre-clinical science journal articles. In addition, it provides links to the full text for many articles. The MeSH search function uses more than 22,000 subject headings that can be combined to narrow the focus and filter out extraneous material. The MeSH headings represent concepts found in the biomedical literature, such as "Hypertension," "Kidney," "Brain Edema," and "Radioactive Waste." MeSH subheadings, such as "adverse effects," "diagnosis," metabolism," and "therapy," can be attached to MeSH headings to describe a specific aspect of a concept, further narrowing the search. Supplementary concepts are mainly drugs or substances, protocols, and rare disease terms. Once the search headings and subheadings are selected, the Boolean operators "AND,"

"OR," and "NOT" can be used to refine the search. The operator AND selects the references that contain both search terms, OR selects the references that contain either search term, and NOT selects the references that contain the first term but not the second term [9]. In general, the Boolean operator AND is most useful for answering specific clinical questions where a number of MeSH headings are combined in order to focus the search. A PubMed MeSH search (Fig. 9.1) using the terms

"Hyperaldosteronism/drug therapy"[MeSH] AND "Spironolactone/therapeutic use"[MeSH] AND "eplerenone"[Supplementary Concept]

yields the same three randomized clinical trials that appeared in the Google search but narrows the field to a much more manageable 26 articles. Note that the same search using the Boolean operator OR (filling in all three circles in Fig. 9.1) would yield an overwhelming 4646 articles! (Further information on using the MeSH database, including tutorials and webinars, is available at: https://www.nlm.nih.gov/mesh/mesh-home.html).

Regardless of the search method, it is important to be as focused and specific as possible with the search terms in

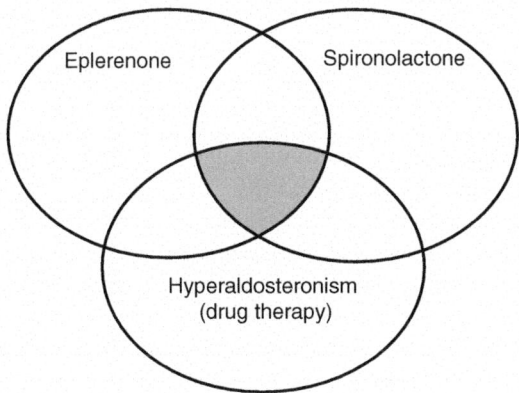

FIGURE 9.1 A PubMed MeSH search using the Boolean operator "AND"

order to capture the important studies while limiting the number of marginally relevant articles. Meanwhile, you can start your patient on spironolactone – which is cheaper ($14.40 vs. $87.90 per month) and at least as effective as eplerenone – and switch to eplerenone if he develops gynecomastia. The cost savings will be $882 per year; you can mention this figure on rounds (see Chap. 10).

Discussing the Literature on Rounds

In medicine, knowledge is power. To cite a pertinent guideline, clinical trial, or case series as you present your patient is the gold standard for the oral case presentation. Researching the literature should become a reflex, especially now that it is so easy to do. When I was a medical student more than 30 years ago, the only way to search the literature was to go to the medical library, page through a gigantic tome called the *Index Medicus*, wander through the stacks to find the article, and then photocopy it. For articles from secondary journals such as the *Korean Journal of Parasitology* or the *Southern African Journal of HIV Medicine*, we would fill out a call slip for the librarian and wait a week or two for a fuzzy faxed copy of the article. Now, amazingly, we have the world's literature instantly available on our smartphones. When I was attending a few weeks ago, I mentioned collagenous colitis in the differential for a middle-aged man with chronic diarrhea. As I turned to go into his room, I saw that my student and intern already had their phones out and knew that they were reading about collagenous colitis.

Your assignment is to access the relevant evidence, discuss it on rounds, and use it to optimize your patient's care. If you fail to search the literature, or decide not to discuss your findings, you might have missed an opportunity to help. I think that students often feel that the team is too busy, or their own oral presentations are already too long, to discuss the results of their literature search. The solution is structural: *make the literature search an integral part of your assessment.* For the patient with primary hyperaldosteronism:

> He needs to be started on an aldosterone antagonist for his hypertension. I searched the literature and found three randomized clinical trials; in one, spironolactone had superior efficacy for hypertension, and in the other two both drugs were equally effective. The cost for spironolactone is $14.40 per month; for eplerenone it is $87.90 per month. I think we should start him on spironolactone 50 mg daily and titrate the dose upward as needed to control his blood pressure. If he develops gynecomastia, we can switch to eplerenone.

Once you have begun presenting your patients in this way, you will find it hard not to incorporate some aspect of your literature search into every case presentation. Finding the best evidence can become a habit – an excellent habit for medical students who want to learn, excel, and provide outstanding care for their patients.

References

1. Katzenstein A. Diagnostic features and differential diagnosis of Churg-Strauss syndrome in the lung. A review. Am J Clin Pathol. 2000;114(5):767–72.
2. Zidan J, Haim N, Beny A, Stein M, Gez E, Kuten A. Octreotide in the treatment of severe chemotherapy-induced diarrhea. Ann Oncol. 2001;12(2):227–9.
3. Fabozzi SJ, Schellhammer PF, el-Mahdi AM. Pulmonary metastases from prostate cancer. Cancer. 1995;75(11):2706–9.
4. Packer CD. The MEDLINE search as a diagnostic maneuver. Arch Intern Med. 2005;165(6):703–4.
5. Parthasarathy HK, Ménard J, White WB, Young WF Jr, Williams GH, Williams B, et al. A double-blind, randomized study comparing the antihypertensive effect of eplerenone and spironolactone in patients with hypertension and evidence of primary aldosteronism. J Hypertens. 2011;29(5):980–90.
6. Karagiannis A, Tziomalos K, Papageorgiou A, Kakafika AI, Pagourelias ED, Anagnostis P, et al. Spironolactone versus eplerenone for the treatment of idiopathic hyperaldosteronism. Expert Opin Pharmacother. 2008;9(4):509–15.

7. Karashima S, Yoneda T, Kometani M, Ohe M, Mori S, Sawamura T, et al. Comparison of eplerenone and spironolactone for the treatment of primary aldosteronism. Hypertens Res. 2016;39(3):133–7.
8. Al-Ubaydli M. Using search engines to find online medical information. PLoS Med. 2005;2(9):e228.
9. Ebbert JO, Dupras DM, Erwin PJ. Searching the medical literature using PubMed: a tutorial. Mayo Clin Proc. 2003;78(1):87–91.

Chapter 10
Adding Value to the Oral Presentation

The Importance of High-Value Care

To understand the importance of high-value, cost-conscious medical care, consider the US healthcare system. Although we pride ourselves on delivering the best medical care in the world, the rapid growth in healthcare costs has led to financial hardship for many Americans. As the cost of care has risen, there has been no consistent improvement in overall quality of care [1], and important measures of quality such as infant mortality rates and life expectancy have not improved despite ever-increasing healthcare spending [2]. Figure 10.1 shows worldwide healthcare spending per capita versus life expectancy in 2013. The outlier is the USA, which spends far more per capita than any other industrialized nation, yet lags behind most of them in life expectancy. Clearly, there is significant waste and overtreatment in the US healthcare system. Unnecessary spending has been estimated at a staggering $750 billion per year [3]. If we are to rein in this unrestrained spending, we must first understand why it is happening and then try to define the values and behaviors that can change the culture.

© Springer Nature Switzerland AG 2019   127
C. D. Packer, *Presenting Your Case*,
https://doi.org/10.1007/978-3-030-13792-2_10

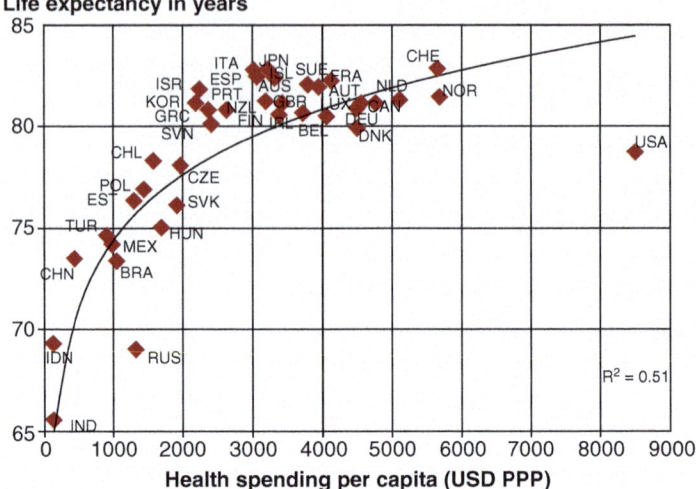

FIGURE 10.1 Health spending per capita versus life expectancy (2013). (Reprinted with permission from OECD Health Statistics 2013; World Bank for non-OECD countries)

Ten Reasons for Overuse

1. *How we are taught.* Medical students and residents practice as they are taught [4]. If they are not trained to avoid overtesting and overtreatment, they are unlikely to change in their future practices.
2. *Prices are opaque.* Physicians are often off by an order of magnitude in their estimates of the costs of tests, procedures, and hospitalizations [5].
3. *Personal risk aversion.* Physicians frequently order unnecessary tests because of a perceived need to protect themselves from risk for malpractice litigation ("fear of missing something").
4. *Preemptive ordering.* This is the so-called shotgun approach, ordering a long list of tests at the outset with little thought about how the results might change management [6].

5. *Demonstrating thoughtfulness*. This applies especially to physicians-in-training, who might order expensive tests for rare or clinically unlikely diseases, just to show that they are considering a broad differential diagnosis.
6. *Hospital myopia*. The practice of ignoring lab and imaging results from an outside hospital and insisting that all tests be repeated in the physician's own hospital. Physicians may rationalize that they are too busy to take the time to request results from the outside hospital or that they need all tests from their own lab "for the sake of consistency."
7. *Redundant ordering*. Ordering tests that have already been ordered by others. This is preventable with a few minutes of chart review before entering new orders; consultants are often the culprits here.
8. *Inertia*. The daily lab and x-ray orders that continue even when the patient is stable and awaiting discharge or transfer.
9. *Patient requests*. Some physicians find it difficult to refuse when patients ask for specific tests, such as MRIs for back pain or chest x-rays when they have a chest cold. This problem has been aggravated by the proliferation of medical information on the Internet, which has expanded the menu for inappropriate test requests.
10. *Lack of trainee feedback about test ordering*. Before ordering any test, whether a CBC or a PET scan, trainees should be taught to ask themselves if the results will change their management of the case. If not, the test should not be ordered. Attending physicians need to stress this simple but important rule for test ordering.

Changing the Culture with High-Value Care

In order to change the culture of unrestrained medical spending, a number of major US medical professional groups and medical educators have developed programs to teach and promote the concept of high-value care. A high-value treatment is when the benefits – **improves outcomes, changes**

management, and meets patient's goals – outweigh the risks – **harm to the patient, cost to the patient, and cost to the system**. The essential goal of high-value care is to improve patient outcomes while decreasing unnecessary healthcare costs and harms. The most robust high-value care program to date is the American College of Physicians' well-publicized "Choosing Wisely" campaign [7]. The Choosing Wisely lists ("Things Providers and Patients Should Question") give specific, evidence-based recommendations across a wide range of specialties that physicians and patients can use to help make decisions using high-value care principles. For example:

1. Don't obtain screening exercise electrocardiogram testing in individuals who are asymptomatic and at low risk for coronary heart disease.
2. Don't obtain imaging studies in patients with non-specific low back pain.
3. In the evaluation of simple syncope and a normal neurologic examination, don't obtain brain imaging studies (CT or MRI).
4. In patients with low pretest probability of venous thromboembolism, obtain a high-sensitive D-dimer measurement as the initial diagnostic test; don't obtain imaging studies as the initial diagnostic test [7].

Training medical students to practice (and teach) high-value care principles is imperative if we are to control healthcare spending and improve quality in the long run. Medical students are a malleable and receptive audience; they have not yet formed their testing and spending habits. A strong high-value care curriculum across US medical schools could lead to substantial cost savings and quality improvement in the long run.

Although medical students may be reluctant at first to discuss cost issues when they present their patients, there is evidence that they are able to identify wasteful practices and even propose practical solutions [8]. A simple and repeatable method for incorporating high-value care into the oral case presentation would help to increase student confidence and normalize discussions of value on rounds and in the clinic.

SOAP-V: Adding Value to the Oral Presentation

SOAP-V (Subjective-Objective-Assessment-Plan-Value) is a new tool that medical students can use to add a discussion of value to their oral presentations and written notes [9, 10]. SOAP-V adds V for value to the traditional SOAP format. It prompts students to consider three questions to evaluate and justify the proposed testing and treatment plan:

1. *Evidence of value.* Before ordering a test, have you and the team considered whether the result would change management? Before ordering a treatment, have you considered the evidence for the treatment vs. no treatment or an alternative treatment?
2. *Patient values.* Have you discussed with the patient their goals and values? Do they recognize the potential harm of the test/treatment compared to alternatives?
3. *Relative cost.* What is the approximate cost of the test/treatment? Are there less costly alternatives with similar benefits?

A CBC is unlikely to change management in a patient who is 72 hours out from an upper GI bleed, with stable vital signs and no further evidence of bleeding. An 82-year-old man with congestive heart failure will not benefit from a screening colonoscopy. A 62-year-old woman in the ICU with cholecystitis and sepsis might be better managed with a cholecystostomy rather than a cholecystectomy. These are situations that should trigger **evidence of value** discussions in your oral presentation. Sometimes these discussions require a literature search, a review of guidelines, and an understanding of pretest probabilities and Bayes theorem; sometimes all that's required is a sense of the big picture and some good common sense.

Assessment of **patient values** means sitting down with your patients and trying to understand their goals and values, with specific reference to the tests and procedures that have been proposed for them. A woman with abdominal pain is very concerned about the cost of a CT scan and would prefer not to have it if possible. A man with stage IV lung cancer who has been admitted for a restaging PET scan and a liver biopsy might be ready to talk about hospice care. These conversations are critical components of SOAP-V and of high-value care in general; without dialogue and shared decision-making, high-value care becomes little more than an evidence-based medicine accounting exercise.

Estimation of the **relative cost** of tests or treatments requires both knowledge of potential alternatives that might be less costly and a reliable way to estimate the cost of any test, procedure, or hospitalization. For example, consider the question of follow-up imaging for kidney stones. It has been shown that if the kidney stone is visible on the scout film of the initial CT scan, it is radiopaque and will also be seen on a KUB (kidney, ureter, and bladder) abdominal x-ray. In one study, it was determined that KUB could be used for follow-up instead of a repeat CT scan in 63% of cases [11]. According to healthcarebluebook.com, a free guide that provides fair prices for healthcare services [12], the price for an abdominal x-ray is $52, and the price for a non-contrast abdominal CT is $760. In addition, an abdominal CT results in significantly more radiation exposure than a KUB and a higher likelihood of incidental findings that could lead to unnecessary imaging and invasive procedures. Thus, the immediate and down-stream costs and potential harms of a CT scan for kidney stone follow-up are substantially higher than with a KUB. In view of the increasing incidence and prevalence of nephrolithiasis worldwide, the potential cost savings with KUB follow-up in appropriate cases could be considerable.

A number of US medical schools have adopted SOAP-V and provide their students with a card (Fig. 10.2) that gives the elements of the SOAP note; the questions to consider for evidence of value, patient values, and relative cost; and the

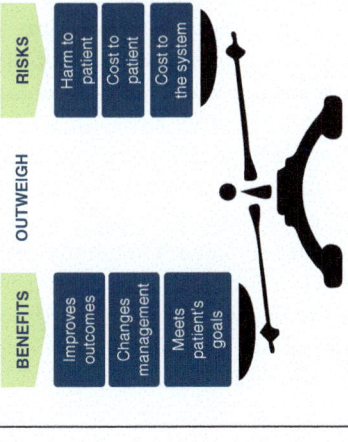

FIGURE 10.2 SOAP-V for presentations or notes [10]. (Reprinted from Moser et al. [10], Copyright 2017, with permission from Elsevier)

link to healthcarebluebok.com for cost information. Armed with this useful card, medical students should be ready to discuss value...but when should it be brought up and how should it be presented?

When to Discuss Value

High-value care can be discussed at any time – before rounds, after rounds, early in the morning, or late at night – whenever a test or procedure is proposed. The best time, however, is usually during the oral presentation, as part of the assessment and plan. This is true for all new admissions, especially transfer patients, who often receive low value care because of hospital myopia and redundant testing (see Chap. 3). The same is true for daily SOAP presentations of established patients, where the cost-conscious student can start a discussion about whether more testing will really change management, call out lab-order inertia, and bring the patient's goals and values into the conversation. High-value care can also be discussed in the context of the differential diagnosis, as explained in Chap. 8; following the Law of Sigma – *consider rare or unusual manifestations of the patient's known disease before positing a completely new diagnosis* – usually leads to a more cost-effective work-up, and this can be explicitly discussed while reviewing the differential. For example, in the case of the patient with a seizure disorder presenting with nystagmus, ataxia, and orthostatic hypotension, it makes sense to argue for a $34 phenytoin level *before* ordering a $969 MRI of the brain...and the dollar numbers need to be a part of the discussion! Another time to discuss value is when the student sits down with the intern or resident to write admission orders, which are fraught with the dangers of low value practices such as demonstrating thoughtfulness and preemptive ordering (the "shotgun" approach). Lower cost testing options, patient preferences, and keeping an eye on the big picture can also be part of the discussion when calling consults and conferring with specialists. Finally, though, the most important conversation about value occurs at the bedside, with the patient. Understanding the patient's goals and values is the sine qua non of high-value care.

How to Discuss Value

First of all, students must understand that they do not need to hesitate or apologize when it comes to bringing up cost issues on rounds. These days, everybody is aware of the importance of high-value care, and the best attendings and residents are already talking about it and teaching it. Although it is true that the ethics of high-value care are sometimes contentious [13], anyone who ignores or belittles a student for bringing up value is an embarrassment to the profession. Second, students do not need to discuss all three components of high-value care in every presentation. A simple comment about the patient's preferences, the cost of a test, or the questionable utility of a procedure is often enough to get the value discussion going. Third, students should cite guidelines, randomized trials, and other evidence to support their thinking about the proposed test or procedure; if you think your stable patient with a hemoglobin of 7.4 g/dL does not need a blood transfusion, be prepared to explain why not [14]. Fourth, high-value care should not be an aside or an afterthought. Embed the discussion of value in your assessment and plan. Consider the following examples:

1. The patient is a 59-year-old woman with a left knee meniscal tear diagnosed by MRI last week. The MRI also revealed moderate osteoarthritis. She's having moderate pain with walking, mild swelling, and occasional locking of the knee. Her health insurance has a high deductible, and she would prefer to avoid surgery if possible. The cost of a knee arthroscopy is $3000–5000, and the cost of a full course of physical therapy would be $1000–2000. A randomized controlled trial of patients 45 and over with meniscal tear and mild-to-moderate arthritis showed similar results at 6 and 12 months with surgery or physical

therapy [15]. I think that physical therapy would be a reasonable approach for her, and it would be in keeping with her preference to avoid surgery. We could offer her a corticosteroid knee injection today to reduce the pain and swelling and help her to tolerate the physical therapy.

2. This 63-year-old man was admitted with 3 days of left lower quadrant pain, fever, and leukocytosis and was found to have uncomplicated diverticulitis on CT scan. The latest guidelines recommend only supportive treatment without antibiotics for most patients with uncomplicated acute diverticulitis [16]. In a randomized clinical trial of observation versus antibiotic treatment in more than 500 patients with CT-proven uncomplicated acute diverticulitis, there was no difference in time to recovery, readmission, recurrent diverticulitis, need for sigmoid resection, or mortality, and the observation patients had a significantly shorter length of stay of 2 versus 3 days [17]. The basic science behind this is that acute diverticulitis is now thought to be an inflammatory process rather than bacterial infection with microperforation. In terms of cost savings, subtracting 3 days' treatment with piperacillin-tazobactam ($13.58/dose) and 1 day of hospitalization (at $2143/day for diverticulitis), we would expect to save approximately $2300 by observing and giving supportive treatment without antibiotics. By holding off on unnecessary antibiotics, we also can avoid the risks of allergic reactions, *C. difficile* colitis, and antimicrobial resistance. I propose that we continue observation, give IV hydration and analgesics as needed, and let him eat when his abdominal pain is better.

Soap-V Practice Cases

For additional work on incorporating high-value care in your patient presentations, consider the following cases: a 34-year-old woman with severe low back pain and a 65-year-old man with a heart failure exacerbation. Apply SOAP-V principles to answer the management and testing questions for each case and think about how you might frame the value discussion in your assessment and plan. Use healthcareblue-book.com for cost information. Answers and explanations for both cases are given at the end of the chapter.

Case 1

A 34-year-old woman presents with 5 days of severe low back pain radiating down the side of her right leg to the top of the foot. The pain is excruciating at times. She has no chronic medical problems and no history of back surgery or chronic back pain. She does not recall any trauma, although she had been lifting some heavy boxes earlier on the day the pain started. There is no leg weakness and no fecal or urinary incontinence; no fevers or chills. No history of IV drug use. She has tried OTC ibuprofen for the pain without much relief.

On physical exam, VS 98.4 76 14 122/74. She appears uncomfortable; gait is normal, no foot drop. There is mild lumbar paraspinous spasm and lumbar spinous tenderness at the L4–5 level. Straight leg raise is positive at 30° on the right; contralateral straight leg raise (radicular pain in the right leg with raising the left leg) is also positive. Motor 5/5 and symmetric in both lower extremities; knee and ankle reflexes are 2+ bilaterally. On sensory exam, there is decreased sensation to pinprick in the right L5 distribution.

1. What is your diagnosis?
2. Are any imaging studies needed? Would you order lumbosacral spine films? MRI of the lumbar spine? What are the costs of these studies?
3. What initial treatment would you prescribe?
4. Would you refer her to a spine surgeon or to physical therapy?
5. How would present your assessment and plan for this patient using SOAP-V principles?

(Use healthcarebluebook.com to find costs of the imaging procedures and choosingwisely.org to view recommendations for acute low back pain.)

Case 2

A 65-year-old man with h/o HFrEF (EF 35% on echocardiogram 6 months ago), HTN, and type 2 DM presented to the ER with 1 week of progressive exertional dyspnea, three-pillow orthopnea, paroxysmal nocturnal dyspnea, and bilateral leg edema with a 15 lb weight gain. Over the past week, he had missed several doses of his furosemide and other heart failure medicines and gone out several times for fast food. He has not had any chest pain. A stress test at the time of his heart failure diagnosis 18 months ago was negative for ischemia or myocardial scar.

On physical exam, VS 98.0 96 24 156/92; room air O_2 saturation 91%; JVP 12 cm; lungs with bibasilar rales; heart regular S1S2 with no murmur or gallop; abdomen soft and non-distended, no tenderness, and no masses or hepatosplenomegaly; and legs with 1+ pitting pedal and pretibial edema to mid-calf.

He is treated with furosemide 40 mgIV and diureses 800 cc in 1 hour, with significant improvement in his dyspnea and orthopnea.

1. What additional testing would you order in the ER? See "Heart Failure Worksheet" (Table 10.1). Complete the "Benefit" and "Harm" section for each potential test.
2. Should this patient be hospitalized? What is the average total cost for a heart failure hospitalization?
3. If you opted for outpatient management, what would be your treatment and follow-up plan?
4. How would you present your assessment and plan for this patient using SOAP-V principles?

Answers for SOAP-V Practice Cases

Case 1

1. Acute low back pain with right L5 radiculopathy; possible L5 disc herniation. In the absence of suspicion for malignancy, spinal infection, or significant neurologic findings, imaging is not indicated.

    Costs: LS spine films, $77; MRI of lumbar spine, $540

TABLE 10.1 Heart failure worksheet for SOAP-V practice Case 2 (Complete the "Benefit" and "Harm" section for each test or procedure, and decide which should be ordered for this patient)

Test	Benefit	Harm	Cost (charges)
Troponin			$75.00
CPK			$60.00
CBC			$50.00
Electrolyte panel			$50.00
BNP			$75.00
EKG			$60.00
CXR			$100.00
TTE (echocardiogram)			$1000.00
Stress echo/nuclear stress test			$2000.00
Cardiac catheterization			$8000.00

2. Guidelines from the American College of Emergency Physicians:

Avoid lumbar spine imaging in the emergency department for adults with nontraumatic back pain unless the patient has severe or progressive neurologic deficits or is suspected of having a serious underlying condition (such as vertebral infection, cauda equina syndrome, or cancer with bony metastasis).

American Academy of Family Physicians:

Don't do imaging for low back pain within the first 6 weeks, unless red flags are present. Red flags include, but are not limited to, severe or progressive neurological deficits or when serious underlying conditions such as osteomyelitis are suspected. Imaging of the lower spine before 6 weeks does not improve outcomes, but does increase costs. Low back pain is the fifth most common reason for all physician visits.

3, 4. Conservative treatment is indicated. Medication options include NSAIDs, a short burst of corticosteroids, and gabapentin or amitriptyline for neuropathic pain.

Physical therapy is also helpful for many patients. Early surgical referral is not indicated in the absence of the red flags listed above. Intractable pain after 6 weeks of conservative treatment is an indication for MRI and possible surgical referral. In the long run, 5- and 10-year follow-up studies show no difference in outcomes for conservative versus surgical treatment in patients with lumbar disc herniation.

5. Assessment: A 34-year-old woman with acute low back pain and right L5 radiculopathy. No history of trauma; low suspicion for infection, cancer, or cauda equine syndrome; and no significant neurologic deficits. Imaging is not indicated. No indication for surgical referral at this time. Patient agrees with plan for conservative treatment.

Plan: Prednisone 40 mg daily for 5 days and then start naproxen 500 mg BID prn for pain. Add gabapentin and uptitrate as needed for persistent neuropathic pain. Physical therapy referral. Follow up in 4–6 weeks.

Case 2

1. See "Heart Failure Worksheet" (Table 10.2). This is the preceptor version with benefits and harms of tests completed.
2. Cost of a hospitalization for heart failure: $5590.
3. Outpatient management of uncomplicated heart failure is commonly done after initial treatment in the ER, usually with high-dose po furosemide (or other loop diuretic) given twice daily for the first several days, and clinic follow-up within 5–7 days. Limiting factors for outpatient management include poor patient compliance, mental illness, and unstable social situations such as homelessness.
4. Assessment: A 65-year-old man with HFrEF, HTN, and type 2 DM, presenting with signs and symptoms of moderate volume overload, probably caused by poor compliance with diet and medications over the past week. Low suspicion for ischemia; no evidence of ACS. Renal function is stable; electrolytes are normal. There is no indication for

TABLE 10.2 Completed heart failure worksheet for SOAP-V practice Case 2

Test	Benefit	Harm	Cost (charges)
Troponin	None in absence of suspicion for ACS	False+ or borderline result might lead to unnecessary testing and procedures	$75.00
CPK	Same as for troponin	Same as for troponin	$60.00
CBC	Unlikely to change management without clinical suspicion for anemia or infection	Unnecessary expense	$50.00
Electrolyte panel	Useful to r/o AKI or electrolyte disorder before initiating diuresis		$50.00
BNP	Will not change management	Unnecessary expense	$75.00
EKG	Potentially useful to detect new arrhythmia, conduction disorder, or ischemia		$60.00

(continued)

TABLE 10.2 (continued)

Test	Benefit	Harm	Cost (charges)
CXR	Potentially useful to detect pleural or pericardial effusions, which might change management	Small dose of radiation; incidental findings that may require additional imaging	$100.00
TTE (echocardiogram)	None in absence of suspicion for pericardial tamponade, valvular disease, etc.	Unnecessary expense	$1000.00
Stress echo/ nuclear stress test	None in absence of suspicion for ischemia	Unnecessary expense	$2000.00
Cardiac catheterization	None in absence of STEMI or ACS	Unnecessary expense; risk of complications	$8000.00

repeat stress testing, echocardiogram, or cardiac catheterization. The patient prefers to be discharged to home and states that he understands the importance of better compliance. Discharge with close outpatient follow-up is reasonable given his good response to IV furosemide in the ER.

Plan: Discharge on furosemide 40 mg po BID. Continue other heart failure medicines (lisinopril, metoprolol SR) as before. Home nursing consult for medication teaching and compliance. Follow up with PCP in 5–7 days.

References

1. Hussey PS, Wertheimer S, Mehrotra A. The association between health care quality and cost: a systematic review. Ann Intern Med. 2013;158(1):27–34.
2. Rapaport L. U.S. health spending twice other countries' with worse results. https://www.reuters.com/article/us-health-spending/u-s-health-spending-twice-other-countries-with-worse-results-idUSKCN1GP2YN. Accessed 26 Oct 2018.
3. Institute of Medicine. The healthcare imperative: lowering costs and improving outcomes. Washington, DC: The National Academies Press; 2010.
4. Chen C, Petterson S, Phillips R, Bazemore A, Mullan F. Spending patterns in region of residency training and subsequent expenditures for care provided by practicing physicians for Medicare beneficiaries. JAMA. 2014;312(22):2385–93.
5. Allan GM, Lexchin J. Physician awareness of diagnostic and nondrug therapeutic costs: a systematic review. Int J Technol Assess Health Care. 2008;24(2):158–65.
6. Mendu ML, McAvay G, Lampert R, Stoehr J, Tinetti ME. Yield of diagnostic tests in evaluating syncopal episodes in older patients. Arch Intern Med. 2009;169:1299.
7. http://www.choosingwisely.org/societies/american-college-of-physicians/. Accessed 27 Oct 2018.
8. Tartaglia KM, Kman N, Ledford C. Medical student perceptions of cost-conscious care in an internal medicine clerkship: a thematic analysis. J Gen Intern Med. 2015;30(10):1491–6.
9. Moser EM, Huang G, Packer CD, Glod S, Smith CD, Alguire PC, et al. SOAP-V: introducing a method to empower medical students as change agents in bending the cost curve. J Hosp Med. 2016;11(3):217–20.
10. Moser EM, Fazio S, Packer CD, Glod SA, Smith CD, Alguire PC, et al. SOAP to SOAP-V: a new paradigm for teaching students high value care. Am J Med. 2017;130(11):1331–6.
11. Johnston R, Lin A, Du J, Mark S. Comparison of kidney-ureter-bladder abdominal radiography and computed tomography scout films for identifying renal calculi. BJU Int. 2009;104(5):670–3.
12. Healthcare Bluebook. https://www.healthcarebluebook.com/ui/consumerfront. Accessed 2 Nov 2018.
13. DeCamp M, Tilburt JC. Ethics and high-value care. J Med Ethics. 2017;43(5):307–9.

14. Carson JL, Guyatt G, Heddle NM, Grossman BJ, Cohn CS, Fung MK, et al. Clinical practice guidelines from the AABB: red blood cell transfusion thresholds and storage. JAMA. 2016;316(19):2025–35.
15. Katz JN, Brophy RH, Chaisson CE, de Chaves L, Cole BJ, Dahm DL, et al. Surgery versus physical therapy for a meniscal tear and osteoarthritis. N Engl J Med. 2013;368:1675–84.
16. Carabotti M, Annibale B. Treatment of diverticular disease: an update on latest evidence and clinical implications. Drugs Context. 2018;7:212526.
17. Daniels L, Unlu C, de Korte N, van Dieren S, Stockmann HB, Vrouenraets BC, et al. Randomized clinical trial of observational versus antibiotic treatment for a first episode of CT-proven uncomplicated acute diverticulitis. Br J Surg. 2017;104(1):52–61.

Chapter 11
Teaching Rounds: Speaking Up, Getting Involved, and Learning to Accept Uncertainty

Teaching Rounds: The Student's Role

I'm always happy when medical students speak up and get involved in the discussion during teaching rounds. They are taking advantage of a tremendous learning opportunity. Nowhere else can a student hear a practical discussion of the natural history, pathophysiology, diagnosis, and treatment of 10 or 12 diseases, listen as the patients describe their symptoms, and observe the key physical exam findings at the bedside – all in the space of a couple of hours on morning rounds! In 6 weeks, a typical student might admit and present 18–20 patients on rounds and see and hear about more than 100 others. Sometimes my students complain that there isn't enough time in the clerkship to do the hundreds of multiple-choice review questions they think they need for their shelf and board exams. In my opinion, there is no better test prep or board review than paying careful attention to what is happening every morning on teaching rounds and then taking a few minutes every night to read about the day's patients.

Teaching rounds (also known as attending rounds) combine teaching and patient care. The proportion of teaching

C. D. Packer, *Presenting Your Case*,
https://doi.org/10.1007/978-3-030-13792-2_11

time on rounds depends on how busy the team is – the number of patients, how sick they are – and the attending's level of interest in teaching. Teaching may occur in the conference room, in the hallway outside the patient's room, and at the bedside. Bedside teaching is particularly important, because some things – especially physical examination findings – can only be taught at the bedside. Also, even in our age of "techno-medicine" [1], there are still many diagnoses that can only be made at the bedside, such as cellulitis, herpes zoster, Parkinson's disease, rheumatoid arthritis, and a host of others (especially neurologic, rheumatologic, and ophthalmologic diseases) [2]. Some think that bedside teaching is a dying art, due to many factors such as resident physician duty hour limits, medical record documentation requirements, shorter lengths of hospital stays, and sophisticated diagnostic technologies [3]. Paradoxically, however, I think that technology will help to revive bedside teaching. I have seen the terrific teaching that our young hospitalist attendings are doing with bedside ultrasound to assess volume status, cardiac function, presence of ascites, etc., and to guide procedures such as paracentesis and thoracentesis. In 10 years, all medical students will carry personal ultrasound devices; in 20 years, I think that ultrasound will replace the stethoscope.

Good teachers expect a response to their efforts. In fact, the most important part of medical teaching is often the back-and-forth, Socratic dialogue that ensues after an interesting observation or an unusual physical finding. In the following scenario, an attending engages his student in a discussion of the hormonal response to heart failure as a way to explain the relationship between heart failure and hyponatremia. The student applies her basic science knowledge and thinks well on her feet, with some gentle guidance from the attending. Note that the attending finishes the discussion with a teaching point:

Attending: Why do you think our patient with acute decompensated heart failure has hyponatremia?

Student: I'm not sure…

Attending:	Well, think about it this way. What's happening with his cardiac output?
Student:	It's low, of course.
Attending:	And how has his blood pressure been running?
Student:	Mostly in the 90's systolic, around 95/60.
Attending:	Right. So although he has edema and extravascular volume overload, how is his circulating blood volume?
Student:	I think…it's low.
Attending:	And what is the hormonal compensation for low intravascular volume and low blood pressure?
Student:	Well, the renin/angiotensin/aldosterone axis is activated, which maintains volume by increasing renal sodium reabsorption in the kidneys. And catecholamine levels are high, which causes vasoconstriction and tachycardia…and I think increased sympathetic tone also increases sodium reabsorption.
Attending:	Excellent. And what happens when the cardiac baroreceptors sense low blood volume and low blood pressure? It's a posterior pituitary hormone…
Student:	Vasopressin?
Attending:	Yes! Arginine vasopressin levels spike when the baroreceptors sense low pressure. How could this cause hyponatremia?
Student:	Vasopressin causes increased water absorption in the kidneys. It concentrates the urine and dilutes the plasma…which causes hyponatremia.
Attending:	Exactly. And hyponatremia is well known to be a marker for increased mortality in heart failure. The lower the sodium, the worse the prognosis. [4]

Another way to get involved is to ask questions on rounds. Good teachers want to know what their students are thinking. Students who ask questions are perceived as engaged, thoughtful, and curious. Note that the questions do not necessarily need to be "deep" or profound. Asking straightforward technical and management questions can stimulate useful discussion:

> When you percuss the liver, why do you keep your fingers parallel to the liver margin?
> Why did you say that a history of sulfa allergy is important when we're thinking of starting a patient on hydrochlorothiazide [5]?
> I'm not clear on why ciprofloxacin would not be the first choice for empiric coverage for a urinary tract infection [6]?
> Why did you ask our elderly patient with a lifelong goiter where he was born and raised [7]?

Another great way to contribute on rounds is to bring the discussion around to the big picture. Let's say, for example, that you are caring for a 74-year-old man with moderately severe dementia who was admitted with heart failure and subsequently found to have severe aortic stenosis. The team is focused on the preoperative work-up and has decided that a transcatheter aortic valve replacement (TAVR) would be the preferred option. The resident is anxious to go ahead with the TAVR procedure now that the patient's heart failure has been optimized. The patient is unable to understand the reason for the procedure or give consent; he states that his heart is "fine."

Resident: So it looks like we can arrange to have the TAVR done as soon as tomorrow.

Attending: The patient lacks capacity. We'll need to get consent from his daughter – she has power of attorney for his health care decisions.

Student: I spoke about it with her last night. She's ambivalent about a valve replacement procedure for her father; she wants him to live, but worries that he'll undergo pain and suffering without understanding the reason for it. She is also concerned about the expense of the procedure, that his savings will be exhausted and there will be no money left for his long-term dementia care.

Attending: It sounds like we need to talk more about this. Let's set up a family conference. We should ask his geriatrician to attend…and maybe somebody from the Ethics Committee as well.

Student: I also did a literature search on TAVR outcomes in patients with dementia. The PARTNER Trial from 2014 showed that decreased cognition is one of the risk factors for poor outcomes (death or poor quality of life) at one, six, and 12 months [8]. It seems to me that given his advanced dementia, this patient's prognosis is poor with or without the TAVR procedure.

Attending: That's extremely helpful. It needs to be part of the discussion at the family conference tomorrow.

Teaching rounds is also an excellent time for patient advocacy. If your patient is in pain, or anxious, or confused about the plan of care, these issues should be brought up and addressed on rounds. If your patient is homeless and you're concerned that his discharge plans are inadequate to ensure good follow-up, talk about it on rounds. If your patient's husband died 3 months ago and you're worried that her deep bereavement might make her unable to handle a complex treatment regimen, propose a simpler one on rounds. Contrary to what some students believe, the educational value of these simple humanistic interventions can be considerable. Physicians treat pain, allay anxiety, and work to make the "externals cooperate" (as Hippocrates put it) every day of their professional lives. This is the art of medicine, the *ars longa*, the heart of medical practice. Learning and discussing the art of medicine on rounds can be one of the most rewarding and inspiring experiences in medical education.

Teaching Decisiveness: A Paradox in Medical Education

Medical students are rightly taught to be cautious, to avoid mistakes, and to understand the mechanisms of medical error. They are frequently reminded that, as students, they are primarily reporters and interpreters rather than decision-makers. As they gain experience on the wards, they note that the complexities of real-life medicine can lead to uncertainty and disagreement on diagnosis and treatment. As they see their attendings and residents grapple daily with uncertainty, many must feel that they are a long way from becoming the confident decision-makers their future patients will need them to be.

When I asked one of my former medical students what he had been taught about decisiveness, he had this thoughtful comment:

> It occurred to me on one of my last rotations that medical students (especially on rounds) are frequently encouraged to take a strong stance and "just act confident about it," even when they have no idea what is going on. On one hand, I understand this is a method to try to compel a student to think through a problem. On the other hand, I think it is part of a surprisingly pervasive culture of medicine that (a) encourages people to act like they know more than they really know and (b) underappreciate uncertainty. I think both of these can be potentially dangerous.

These concerns are well-founded. The last thing we want is to have our students going off half-cocked, making ill-founded and ill-reasoned decisions that would put patients at risk. On the other hand, the practice of medicine demands decisiveness. In my primary care clinic, and when I am attending on the wards, I make dozens of decisions every day. The same is true for every practicing physician. How do we get from the appropriately hesitant student to the reasonably confident attending? Is decisiveness simply a function of time, experience, and assumption of responsibility? Is it a teachable skill or a fixed personality trait?

In the medical education literature, decisiveness per se is rarely mentioned, but there are many studies investigating "tolerance of uncertainty," "tolerance of ambiguity," and "need for cognitive closure." The first two of these are prerequisites for decisiveness, and the third can be a serious barrier. Physicians with intolerance of uncertainty and a high need for cognitive closure have been found to have higher levels of stress, burnout, and therapeutic inertia [9, 10]. Medical students with high tolerance of ambiguity are more inclined to select rural and underserved urban practices, which demand independent decision-making [10, 11]. On the whole, these studies suggest that tolerance of ambiguity and uncertainty is a trait (or coping mechanism?) that physicians develop in order to make the decisions that need to be made without undue stress. Physicians with a strong need for cognitive closure may have more trouble with decisions, less flexibility, and more stress.

Interestingly, tolerance of ambiguity decreases during medical school [12]. This may reflect the student's abrupt third-year transition from the relative certainties of the basic sciences to the strange new alchemy of clinical medicine, where experience and "the art of medicine" hold more sway. Physicians' tolerance of uncertainty appears to be higher than that attributed to them by students [13], which probably reflects a lack of teaching about (or admitting to) uncertainty in our clinical medical education. Perhaps this is why there is no formal "decisiveness" training in medicine: it would expose the faint rim of uncertainty that surrounds most of our medical decisions.

I think that we should discuss decisiveness and acceptance of uncertainty with our students, both formally – in the curriculum – and informally on rounds and in the clinic. As it stands now, most of the discussion centers on statistics: pre- and posttest probabilities, confidence intervals, number needed to treat, Bayesian reasoning, and so forth. Statistics can help to increase confidence and reduce uncertainty, but decisiveness requires more than a low p-value or a high posttest probability. Decisiveness requires experience, nerve, and a sense of what is at stake for the patient.

Since discussions of cognitive closure and acceptance of uncertainty don't necessarily happen on rounds, students should ask questions about how clinical decisions are being made in real time:

Student: I was wondering why we're discharging Mr. Murray today. We don't have a diagnosis yet for his abdominal pain, and it really isn't much better than the day he was admitted.

Attending: Well, he's eating a little better now, and keeping down fluids. He doesn't need the IV any more. I think he's okay to go home.

Student:	But we don't know what's wrong with him!
Attending:	That's true...but we know what's *not* wrong with him. Thanks to our lab work-up and CT scan, we know that he doesn't have cholecystitis, pancreatitis, appendicitis, diverticulitis, bowel obstruction, or nephrolithiasis. There are no signs of ischemic bowel. There's no abdominal aortic aneurysm. We've ruled out the most serious causes of abdominal pain.
Student:	Well, he could have peptic ulcer disease. We haven't done an EGD yet.
Attending:	That's right, but we've started him empirically on a high-dose proton pump inhibitor. If he does have PUD, gastritis, or esophagitis, it should heal up after a few weeks of treatment.
Student:	But what if he has a bad ulcer and it starts to bleed? What if it's gastric cancer?
Attending:	If he bleeds, he'll need to come back to the hospital. If it's gastric cancer, which is unlikely with his normal CT scan, the PPI treatment will not be effective. We'll make sure his PCP sees him in a week or so for follow-up. He can always be readmitted if necessary, or have an EGD later as an outpatient.
Student:	But what's our diagnosis for the discharge summary?
Attending:	Non-specific abdominal pain. He's ready to go home. If there's something serious going on, it will declare itself. If not (which I think is more likely), he'll get better.
Student:	I'm trying to understand. Why not just do the EGD now. Why accept uncertainty?
Attending:	There is some risk as well as expense with an EGD, and it's not clear to me that it would change our management at this point. There's a good chance that this is functional or somatic pain. In one study of 186 patients who were diagnosed with acute non-specific abdominal

pain, over 70% were free of symptoms after 20 years of follow-up [14]. All things considered, I'm comfortable with discharging him today.

This kind of discussion is invaluable to students. It reveals the fact that most medical decisions are probabilistic to some degree and that the day-to-day realities of medical practice require acceptance of uncertainty on a daily and sometimes hourly basis. It also shows that good and rational decisions can be made without full cognitive closure. The paradox is that with decisiveness there needs to be a "letting go" of absolute certainty. Learning to make good decisions while accepting uncertainty is a lot like learning to juggle; it's very hard at first, but when everything comes together it's as natural as breathing.

References

1. Baumgartner F. Human medicine versus techno-medicine. Tex Heart Inst J. 2009;36(3):268–9.
2. McGee S. Bedside teaching rounds reconsidered. JAMA. 2014;311(19):1971–2.
3. Cornia PB. How to teach at the bedside. In: Mookherjee S, Cosgrove EM, editors. Handbook of clinical teaching. Cham: Springer International Publishing; 2016. p. 86.
4. Gheorghiade M, Abraham WT, Albert NM, Gattis Stough W, Greenberg BH, O'Connor CM, et al. Relationship between admission serum sodium concentration and clinical outcomes in patients hospitalized for heart failure: an analysis from the OPTIMIZE-HF registry. Eur Heart J. 2007;28(8):980–8.
5. Phipatanakul W, Adkinson NF. Cross-reactivity between sulfon-amides and loop or thiazide diuretics: is it a theoretical or actual risk? Allergy Clin Immunol Int. 2000;12(1):26–8.
6. Fasugba O, Gardner A, Mitchell BG, Mnatzaganian G. Ciprofloxacin resistance in community- and hospital-acquired Escherichia coli urinary tract infections: a systematic review and meta-analysis of observational studies. BMC Infect Dis. 2015;15:545.
7. Schiel J, Wepfer A. Distributional aspects of endemic goiter in the United States. Econ Geogr. 1976;52(2):116–26.

8. Arnold SV, Reynolds MR, Lei Y, Magnuson EA, Kirtane AJ, Kodali SK, et al. Predictors of poor outcomes after transcatheter aortic valve replacement: results from the PARTNER Trial. Circulation. 2014;129(25):2682–90.

9. Iannello P, Mottini A, Tirelli S, Riva S, Antonietti A. Ambiguity and uncertainty tolerance, need for cognition, and their association with stress. A study among Italian practicing physicians. Med Educ Online. 2017;22(1):1270009.

10. Caulfield M, Andolsek K, Grbic D, Roskovensky L. Ambiguity tolerance of students matriculating to U.S. Medical schools. Acad Med. 2014;89(11):1526–32.

11. Eley DS, Leung JK, Campbell N, Cloninger CR. Tolerance of ambiguity, perfectionism and resilience are associated with personality profiles of medical students oriented to rural practice. Med Teach. 2017;39(5):512–9.

12. Han PKJ, Schupack D, Daggett S, Holt CT, Strout TD. Temporal changes in tolerance of uncertainty among medical students: insights from an exploratory study. Med Educ Online. 2015;20:28285.

13. Schor R, Pilpel D, Benbassat J. Tolerance of uncertainty of medical students and practicing physicians. Med Care. 2000;38(3):272–80.

14. Fagerström A, Miettinen P, Valtola J, Juvonen P, Tarvainen R, Ilves I, et al. Long-term outcome of patients with acute non-specific abdominal pain compared to acute appendicitis: prospective symptom audit after two decades. Acta Chir Belg. 2014;114(1):46–51.

Chapter 12
On Pimping

What Is Pimping?

"Pimping" is when an attending physician puts a resident or medical student on the spot by asking a difficult question on rounds, or a series of questions in the Socratic style. A pimp is a person who solicits customers for prostitutes or brothels; in a broader sense, a pimp is someone who exploits others for personal gain. How this term of opprobrium ever attached itself to a pedagogic technique favored by Plato is unclear [1, 2]. The term seems to have originated in Europe, where it has been traced back as far as seventeenth-century London. In the nineteenth century, the German physician and microbiologist Heinrich Koch famously had a series of *Pümpfrage* or "pump questions" ("pimping" might be a corruption of "pumping") that he used in rapid succession on his teaching rounds. The practice reached North America by the early twentieth century and was documented by Flexner as he observed Osler questioning his students on rounds at Johns Hopkins [3]. When I was a medical student in the 1980s, pimping was still a part of everyday life; we more or less accepted it as a rite of passage. Even now I hear medical students discussing pimping on a fairly regular basis, and before I question a student, I often wonder: "Is he going to think I'm pimping him?"

© Springer Nature Switzerland AG 2019
C. D. Packer, *Presenting Your Case*,
https://doi.org/10.1007/978-3-030-13792-2_12

There is no question that pimping can be a source of terror for some medical students and residents. Samuel O. Thier, chair of medicine at Yale in the 1970s, was such an avid pimper that one of his residents fainted from anxiety prior to a case presentation. This earned Dr. Thier the interesting nickname of Syncope Sam [4]. These days, aggressive pimping is passé, but you still might find a few practitioners of the dark art lurking on the wards.

In his satiric essay, "The Art of Pimping" [5], Brancati gives five categories of "pimp questions," which "should come in rapid succession and should be essentially unanswerable." These types of questions are obnoxious and should not be tolerated by medical students:

1. Arcane points of history. (Who performed the first lumbar puncture?)
2. Teleology and metaphysics. (Why are some organs paired?)
3. Exceedingly broad questions. (What is the differential diagnosis of fever of unknown origin?)
4. Eponyms. (Where does one find the semilunar space of Traube?)
5. Technical points of laboratory research. (How active are leukocyte-activated killer cells with or without interleukin 2 against sarcoma in the mouse model?) [4].

Some medical educators have argued that pimping is bad because it divides students into two groups: heroes who answer the questions right and goats who get them wrong. The concern is that the goats will suffer severe trauma to their self-esteem and that this is no way to teach medicine in our enlightened age of cooperative, collegial, and supportive medical education. The underlying assumption seems to be that testing or probing a student's knowledge and problem-solving ability in real time, with patients and colleagues present, is fundamentally unfair and unreasonable.

An unenlightened response to this argument might be that anyone with a backbone can withstand a little good-natured pimping, which provides fun and recreation for the attending and the rest of the team. More to the point, doctors need to be alert, well-informed, and decisive. They need to think on their feet. Their patients will need to be treated now, not after a preliminary hearing and a holiday recess. A properly pimped student (the pro-pimping argument goes) is stimulated to think through a problem in real time, commit to an answer, and reflect on personal strengths and weaknesses. In reality, however, many students who experience aggressive pimping respond not with self-reflection but with anxiety, frustration, and anger. Furthermore, "questioning with the intent to shame and humiliate the learner" [5] can be viewed as mistreatment, which is a serious issue in medical education.

"Socrates Was Not a Pimp"

A more enlightened response comes from Kost and Chen in their article "Socrates was not a pimp: changing the paradigm of questioning in medical education" [6]. They acknowledge the usefulness of probing students' medical knowledge in real time but argue that pimping is harmful and unprofessional and that alternative questioning techniques should be used for teaching and assessment on rounds. They suggest that attendings (1) examine the purpose of each question they pose to learners, (2) apply historic and modern interpretations of Socratic teaching methods that promote critical thinking skills, and (3) consider adult learning theories to make concrete changes to their questioning practices [6].

While adult learning theory and historic interpretation might be a tall order for many attendings, examining the purpose of a question is a reasonable and attainable goal for all medical teachers. Any question that is directly pertinent to the diagnosis and management of a student's patient – once that patient has been seen and examined by the student – is and ought to be fair game. The question "How are we going to manage this patient's post-herpetic neuralgia?" might be pimping of a sort, if asked before the team on rounds, but it's also part of the work that must be done to treat the patient and educate the student. In another case, it would be quite acceptable for an attending to ask about linitis plastica or Virchow nodes if a student were working up a patient with suspected gastric cancer. It would be unreasonable for the attending to quiz this student on the differential diagnosis for a homonymous hemianopsia or the common etiologies of a type B lactic acidosis.

Consider the difference between benign pimping and malignant pimping. In benign pimping, the questions are reasonable, appropriate to the pimpee's level of training, and pertinent to the patient at hand. In benign pimping, the attending tosses up a few slam-dunk questions as a warm-up and gives helpful hints when the questions get tougher. Malignant pimping begins with the hardest question and ends with stony silence and a supercilious sneer. Benign pimping is about education; malignant pimping is about dominance and preserving the power hierarchy. Consider two scenarios where a medical student is working up a patient with advanced chronic kidney disease, and the case is under discussion on morning rounds:

Attending: So we have a 63-year-old woman with stage V chronic kidney disease who was admitted with shortness of breath, fatigue, and failure to thrive. Is it time to start her on dialysis? What do you think, James?

Student: Well, I'm not sure. She's short of breath with moderate exertion, and she has 1+ pretibial edema, but her lungs are clear and her JVP is normal. Her weight is stable since last month. She's oxygenating well on room air. I don't think she's significantly volume overloaded at this point.

Attending:	That's a nice assessment of her volume status. I agree. Does she have any other indications for dialysis? How are today's lab results?
Student:	Her potassium is a little high at 5.2. She's on furosemide 40 mg daily to keep it under control. Her BUN and creatinine are 54 and 5.3. Her calcium is normal, but the phosphorus is high at 4.9.
Attending:	Is she acidotic?
Student:	Her CO_2 is stable at 22. She's been taking sodium bicarbonate for the past couple of months.
Attending:	So her lab results look pretty stable, with no immediate indications for dialysis. What about her other symptoms?
Student:	Well, they're kind of vague…
Attending:	She tells us she's feeling weak, and her appetite has been poor lately. She's had nausea at times, and some leg cramps. She's also had trouble concentrating at work lately.
Student:	I see what you're getting at. She's probably having some symptoms of uremia.
Attending:	I think so. And uremic symptoms can sometimes be an indication for dialysis even without significant hyperkalemia or acidosis.

Attending:	So we have a 63-year-old woman with stage V chronic kidney disease who was admitted with shortness of breath, fatigue, and failure to thrive. James, what are the indications for dialysis?
Student:	Umm…volume overload?
Attending:	Yes, that's one of them. Is she volume overloaded?
Student:	I don't think so.
Attending:	What else? There are five indications for dialysis. You've given me one.
Student (getting flustered):	Let's see…
Attending:	What could kill her?
Student:	Well…an arrhythmia? An MI?
Attending:	Volume overload, hyperkalemia, acidosis, uremia, and pericarditis. You need to know this. Don't you read about your patients?

Note that the attending in the first scenario uses a series of questions and answers to arrive at a better understanding of the indications for dialysis and how they might apply to the student's patient. The questions are broad and flexible, based on the student's responses, and the mood is collegial. The second attending is fixated on the five indications for dialysis and reacts with hostility when the student can't immediately recall them. In addition to mistreatment, this is a lost learning opportunity.

The Pimper Phenotype

Medical students probably wonder if there are certain traits or characteristics that predict the pimping behavior of their attendings. This was all guesswork until quite recently, when researchers at Johns Hopkins published a study that surveyed internal medicine faculty ward attendings on their questioning styles and attitudes toward pimping [7]. Based on the responses, they developed a numeric "pimping score" and divided the faculty into "pimper" and "non-pimper" phenotypes, with pimpers defined as those with scores in the upper quartile. Faculty who were younger, male, specialists, working in large tertiary medical centers, and with lower quality of life indicators were more likely to have high pimping scores. Interestingly, although 45% of faculty reported some positive attitudes about the value of pimping, only 20% reported that pimping was effective in their own teaching practice. The pimper faculty agreed that "pimping of students or residents is an effective teaching strategy on clinical rounds" and that "being pimped by my teachers helped me learn when I was a medical trainee." Faculty who openly endorsed favorable views about the educational value of pimping had sevenfold higher odds of being characterized as "pimpers" by their pimping scores.

The surprising finding in this study is that the most avid pimpers were young, which goes against the notion that pimping is a vestigial practice kept alive by doctors who learned medicine in the age of the dinosaurs. One wonders if the aggressive pimping was a result of insecurity in these young and relatively unhappy attendings.

Pimping the Pimper: The Art of Pimping Back

A few brave and mischievous souls try to turn the tables on their unsuspecting attendings by pimping back (described by Brancati as "the dreaded 'reverse pimp'") [8]. Sometimes pimping back can be as simple as deflecting questions back at the attending, or responding to pimping questions with related but more difficult questions for the attending to ponder. Occasionally, students will attempt the full-blown reverse pimp, which puts them solidly in the questioning role and transfers the stress and anxiety to the attending. Consider this dialogue between Dr. Osler, the gentle but masterful ward attending, and his wily medical student:

Dr. Osler:	Why is this patient breathing 36 times per minute?
Student:	Well...we found something in his urine.
Dr. Osler:	You found something in his urine that's making him tachypneic?
Student:	Yes, actually. You'll never guess what it is.
Dr. Osler:	OK, let's see. Is it urosepsis?
Student:	Nope. No evidence of a UTI.
Dr. Osler:	Hmmm...high urinary catecholamines with heart failure brought on by a pheochromocytoma-associated hypertensive crisis?...Pulmonary carcinoid with bronchospasm and high urinary 5-HIAA? Am I on the right track?
Student (with rising excitement):	No, sir!
Dr. Osler (matter-of-factly):	Then I'd guess you saw calcium oxalate crystals in the urine, which suggests an ethylene glycol overdose. He's Kussmauling to compensate for the severe metabolic acidosis. Have you confirmed that there's an osmolal gap as well as an anion gap? Have you started 4-methylpyrazole? Have you called the renal service to dialyze him?

| Student (deflated): | Yes to all the above, Dr. Osler. How did you know? |
| Dr. Osler: | I read your admission note before rounds. |

The obvious lesson here is that if the student is going to play games, the attending can play along and cunningly reverse the reverse pimp. The subtle lesson is that a good attending learns to parry the student's questions until the learning has been maximized and then ties it all together with a good teaching point or two. The general laughter that undoubtedly followed Dr. Osler's little confession is good for morale and takes the personal edge off the pimping process.

In Defense of Pimping

Brancati defends pimping – when done right – because it can entertain and teach at the same time, and produce "a feisty esprit de corps among the pimped." To avoid the problems of excessive and distracting roundsmanship, he takes a proactive strategy:

> My own approach is to pull each student and intern aside individually at the start of the rotation to explain the distinction I make between style and substance in patient care and medical education. I emphasize that I will evaluate students and interns based on honesty, thoroughness, and knowledge of medicine relevant to the patients currently under their care, not based on their ability to handle pimp questions. [7]

Psychological safety is a very important precondition for effective and educational pimping. According to Amy Edmondson, "group members feel psychologically safe if they sense interpersonal trust, enjoy mutual respect, feel valued, and are comfortable being themselves because the threats of humiliation and hostility are minimized" [9]. If the milieu is safe and comfortable, students are willing to accept the risk-taking that goes with engaging in Socratic discussions on rounds – provided that the pimping questions are fair, the discussion is open and bidirectional, and the pimper's goal is to educate rather than intimidate.

What do students actually think of pimping? A survey of 11 fourth-year medical students showed that all understood the hierarchical nature of pimping and that attendings and residents use it as a tool to assess students' medical knowledge. And perhaps surprisingly, although some of the students had been subjected to malignant pimping, all 11 "were positive about pimping and its effectiveness as a pedagogical tool" [10]. This is, of course, a very small sample, but it does suggest that students can understand why pimping is done, withstand it, and even appreciate it.

How to Respond to Pimping

1. When you're asked a question on rounds, do your best to answer it. If you don't know the answer, say so. A good attending will try another line of questioning that eventually leads you to the right answer, with helpful teaching along the way.
2. Know your patient well, and read up on the diagnosis and treatment plan. All patient management issues are fair game for questioning on rounds.
3. Understand that as a physician-in-training, you are expected to be able to think on your feet and work through problems in real time. Stay calm, and ask questions if you need help or clarification as you give your thoughts on the case.
4. If you encounter an attending or resident who questions you in a hostile, aggressive, or demeaning manner, stand your ground. Tell them politely but firmly that you don't find their teaching style to be helpful or effective, and ask if they can change their approach. If you find it too difficult to speak up, ask your clerkship director or rotation leader to transfer you to a different team. Passively tolerating a toxic work environment is always a bad idea.

5. Don't be afraid to turn the tables and reverse-pimp your attending. Great discussions can happen when the hierarchy is suspended and the questions flow freely in both directions!

References

1. Stanton C, Pierach CA, Kleinman JG, Rustin TA, Brancati FL. Pimper pimped. JAMA. 1989;262(18):2541–2.
2. Brancati FL. Pimping: in reply. JAMA. 1990;263(12):1633.
3. Detsky AS. The art of pimping. JAMA. 2009;301(13):1379–81.
4. Ausiello DA. Introduction of Samuel O. Their, MD. J Clin Invest. 2008;118:3805–10.
5. Brancati FL. The art of pimping. JAMA. 1989;262(1):89–90.
6. Kost A, Chen FM. Socrates was not a pimp: changing the paradigm of questioning in medical education. Acad Med. 2015;90(1):20–4.
7. McEvoy JW, Shatzer JH, Desai SV, Wright SM. Questioning style and pimping in clinical education: a quantitative score derived from a survey of internal medicine teaching faculty. Teach Learn Med. 2019;31(1):53–64.
8. Brancati FL. Pimper pimped: in reply. JAMA. 1989;262(18):2542.
9. Stoddard HA, O'Dell DV. Would Socrates have actually used the "Socratic Method" for clinical teaching? J Gen Intern Med. 2016;31(9):1092–6.
10. Wear D, Kokinova M, Keck-McNulty C, Aultman J. Pimping: perspectives of 4th year medical students. Teach Learn Med. 2006;18(1):87.

Chapter 13
The Art of the 5-Minute Talk

How to Become a "Student-Educator"

As they begin their third-year clinical clerkships, medical students are facing the steepest learning curve (with the possible exception of internship) that they will ever encounter. With all that they are struggling to learn – history-taking, case presentation, differential diagnosis, and an ever-increasing flood of clinical information – it seems almost gratuitous to expect them to be educators as well. Nevertheless, most attendings and residents do expect their students to teach, especially in the form of short, focused talks addressing questions that arise on rounds. Students who are able to research a topic quickly and present a clear and concise 5-minute talk that helps with patient care earn kudos from their teams. Moreover, nothing enhances learning quite like teaching, which requires mastery of the material and careful thought about its implications. Students who provide frequent small aliquots of teaching learn a great deal and also build confidence in their teaching skills.

Why the 5-minute talk? Two minutes is barely enough time to scrape the surface of any topic; 10 minutes exceeds the attention span of most interns, who tend to start typing in orders on their keyboards around the 6-minute mark.

© Springer Nature Switzerland AG 2019
C. D. Packer, *Presenting Your Case*,
https://doi.org/10.1007/978-3-030-13792-2_13

Five minutes is just enough time to answer a focused clinical question, summarize an article, or present a case vignette while keeping the audience fresh and engaged. The 5-minute talk takes very little time away from the busy work day and provides answers to relevant clinical questions that can improve patient care.

The 5-minute talk demands conciseness, organization, and clear thinking. Consider the following recommendations as you plan and research your presentation:

Narrow the Scope

Topics such as "COPD" or "heart failure" are far too broad for a short talk. It's important to narrow the scope by finding a relevant clinical question that needs to be answered. Let's suppose that you have a patient admitted a few days ago with a COPD exacerbation who is now improving and expected to go home soon. The question of whether he should be discharged on a long or short corticosteroid taper was brought up on rounds; this is a perfect topic for a 5-minute talk. In addition, you notice that the patient had not been prescribed a long-acting bronchodilator (LABD) prior to admission, although his FEV1 was only 52% predicted on a recent spirometry. Should he be discharged on budesonide/formoterol or tiotropium? Indications for starting LABDs in COPD would be another good topic for a talk. Finally, thinking a little outside the box, a short talk on the unexpected benefits of beta-blockers (decreased overall mortality, reduced risk of exacerbations) in patients with COPD [1] could provoke some lively discussion. Table 13.1 gives subject areas that are too broad for a 5-minute talk, along with focused, clinically relevant topics that could be covered very well in 5 min. Resist the temptation to tell everything you know about COPD or heart failure. The key to developing a good short talk is to maintain a laser-like focus on the specific clinical question that you think needs to be answered.

TABLE 13.1 Examples of focused, clinically relevant topics for 5-minute talks

Too broad...	Focused, clinically relevant topics
COPD	Short vs. long corticosteroid tapers for COPD exacerbations
	When to start long-acting bronchodilators
	Possible benefits of beta-blockers in severe COPD
CHF	Use of spironolactone in heart failure
	Tachycardia-induced cardiomyopathy
	Indications for left ventricular assist devices
Type 2 diabetes mellitus	Recognizing and treating ketosis-prone type 2 diabetes
	Indications for DPP-4 inhibitors
	Relationship between sulfonylurea treatment and fatty liver
Atrial fibrillation	Rate control vs. rhythm control
	Applying the CHADS-2 score in atrial fibrillation
	Indications for amiodarone
Acute kidney injury	Clinical and pathologic features of acute tubular necrosis
	Use of the FENA and FEUrea in diagnosing AKI
	Significance of eosinophilia in AKI
Anemia	Stages of iron deficiency anemia
	Interpreting the MCV and RDW
	Significance of schistocytes in acute anemia

(continued)

TABLE 13.1 (continued)

Too broad...	Focused, clinically relevant topics
Management of Cirrhosis	Abstinence from alcohol
	Surveillance for varices
	Use of beta-blockers in cirrhosis
	Use of diuretics in cirrhosis
	Drugs to prevent and treat hepatic encephalopathy
	Large-volume paracentesis
	Albumin, midodrine, and octreotide for hepatorenal syndrome
	Transjugular intrahepatic portosystemic shunt (TIPS procedure)

Dig Deep

When you research a clinical question, it's extremely important to dig deep to fully understand the context of the question and the areas of debate and uncertainty. For example, let's say that you are preparing a patient for major surgery and wonder if beta-blocker treatment might reduce the risk of cardiac complications. A superficial review of the literature on perioperative beta-blockers suggests only that there are insufficient data on efficacy and safety to recommend their routine use. A deeper look reveals a tangled history of beta-blocker studies, with one randomized controlled trial (POISE) marred by a major overtreatment effect, and two RCTs (DECREASE-I and DECREASE-IV) that showed dramatic risk reduction with beta-blockers but were tainted by serious academic irregularities [2]. The pros and cons of perioperative beta-blockade should be considered for each patient while we wait for better evidence [3]. On the question of the duration of corticosteroid treatment for COPD exacerbations, recent studies have shown no difference in rehospitalization, reintubation, and 6-month reexacerbation rates with a 5-day versus a 14-day treatment regimen [4, 5]. The 5-day regimen allows for a significant reduction in corticosteroid exposure without increased risk of treatment failure. The key here is the consistency of these findings across several clinical studies; a deep dive into the literature shows very strong evidence for the 5-day regimen.

Digging deep also means considering the implications and downstream effects of a clinical decision or recommendation. For instance, left ventricular assist devices (LVADs) are indicated both as a bridge to transplant and as "destination therapy" in patients with end-stage heart failure. Although these devices can improve quality of life, patients and physicians must understand that there is a very high risk of complications including major bleeding, infection, pump thrombosis, right heart failure, device malfunction, and stroke [6]. Some patients with end-stage heart failure prefer to focus on comfort and palliation rather than accept the risks, burdens, and uncertain benefits of LVAD implantation. Any talk on the use of LVADs in heart failure must go beyond survival statistics and examine some aspects of the patient experience with these devices.

Cite Key Studies

Use the PubMed MeSH search (as described in Chap. 9) to find the clinical trials, guidelines, and other evidence required to answer your clinical question. If randomized controlled trials are lacking, other pertinent forms of evidence, such as cohort and case-control studies, case series, and case reports, should be discussed and evaluated in your talk. Classic studies are great to cite in these short talks. For example, if you have a patient with recently diagnosed colon cancer who presents with a right leg DVT, it's important to discuss the CLOT Trial (2003), which was the first to show that low-molecular-weight heparin is superior to warfarin in preventing recurrent venous thromboembolism in the setting of malignancy [7]. If you admit a patient with acute decompensated heart failure and an ejection fraction of 30%, you can cite the RALES Trial (1999), which showed that adding 25 mg of spironolactone to standard therapy reduces all-cause mortality in heart failure patients with an ejection fraction <35% [8]. Beyond their importance in optimizing patient care, classic trials such as CLOT and RALES stand as important markers on the timeline of modern medical progress and should be familiar to all literate physicians. A short talk with a strong teaching point and a concise review of a classic article is 5 minutes well spent!

Write an Outline

Too much detail can easily sink a 5-minute talk. Information is good, but too much information can be deadly. The best way to avoid overexplanation is to write an outline that keeps your talk focused on the main teaching points. For example, in a talk on the use of diuretics in the management of cirrhosis with ascites, your main points might be:

- Indications for diuretic treatment in cirrhosis with ascites
- Importance of low-sodium diet with diuretic treatment
- Loop diuretics alone are less effective in hypoalbuminemic states – protein-binding is required for transport to the proximal convoluted tubule
- Spironolactone more effective – no protein binding needed, anti-aldosterone effects
- Importance of the 5:2 spironolactone: furosemide ratio in maintaining potassium homeostasis
- Dangers of overdiuresis: hepatorenal syndrome
- How these recommendations apply to our patient

Reference: Pedersen et al. [10].

Each of these six main teaching points can be concisely explained in a minute or less, which keeps you close to the 5-minute target. At the end, it's always useful to comment briefly on how your findings apply to the patient: "He has responded well to spironolactone 100 mg and furosemide 40 mg daily, and his potassium has stayed in the normal range. With diuretic treatment, his ascites has not recurred after the initial large-volume paracentesis last week. He seems to have diuretic-responsive ascites." Finally, the reference, in this case a review article, gives interested team members an opportunity to review the subject in more depth.

Here is an outline for a 5-minute talk on the use of gabapentin for the treatment of alcohol withdrawal, as an alternative to benzodiazepines. The first randomized, double-blind trial to compare gabapentin and lorazepam [9] is cited and discussed:

- Disadvantages of benzodiazepines for alcohol withdrawal: sedation, cognitive impairment, respiratory depression, abuse potential
- Gabapentin mechanism of action: GABAnergic, reverses the low GABA/high glutamate state found after cessation of drinking; normalizes the hyperactive state of the brain that is characteristic of alcohol withdrawal
- Advantages of gabapentin: less sedation, less craving for alcohol, no hepatic metabolism, excreted unchanged in the urine, moderate side-effect profile

From Myrick et al. [9]:

- Randomized, double-blind trial with 100 patients
- Lorazepam vs. high- or intermediate-dose gabapentin for outpatient alcohol withdrawal
- Severity of alcohol withdrawal was measured by the CIWA-Ar over 12 days; alcohol use monitored by verbal report and breath alcohol levels
- CIWA-Ar scores decreased over time in all groups; high-dose gabapentin was statistically superior ($p = 0.009$) but clinically similar to lorazepam (Fig. 13.1)
- Gabapentin patients had lower probability of drinking during treatment and post-treatment periods
- Gabapentin groups also had less craving, anxiety, and sedation compared to lorazepam
- Our hospital has instituted a CIWA-based gabapentin protocol (handout)

Keep It Relevant to Patient Care

Once you have researched a clinical question and presented your findings, apply what you have learned to your patient's case. For example, if your patient had a 14-day corticosteroid taper for his most recent COPD exacerbation, it would be reasonable – based on excellent evidence – to switch him to a 5-day regimen for this hospitalization. On the other hand, if he had been rehospitalized for COPD twice in the past 6 weeks after 5-day prednisone bursts, you might acknowledge the research but argue that your patient's case might require a 14-day course based on his two treatment failures with the 5-day regimen. The point is that randomized trials and guidelines apply to populations, but not necessarily to every individual patient. Don't overlook the uniqueness of your patient.

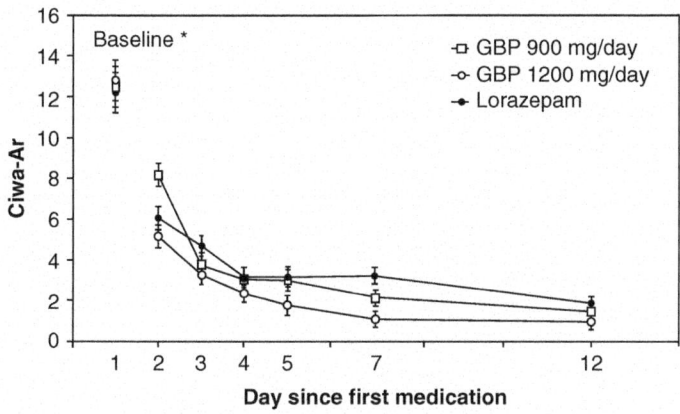

FIGURE 13.1 CIWA-Ar alcohol withdrawal symptom scores over 12 days of treatment with lorazepam and gabapentin. (Republished with permission of John Wiley and Sons Inc., from Myrick et al. [9] permission conveyed through Copyright Clearance Center, Inc.)

Summarize Your Findings in a One-Page Handout

Distribute a concise, one-page handout that summarizes the main points of your 5-minute talk. To keep things simple and avoid unnecessary effort, use your outline (with editing as needed) for the summary handout. Be sure to include any key figures or tables from the studies you cited in your talk.

A summary helps to solidify the main teaching points and shows consideration and respect for the other members of the team. It also serves as a tangible reminder of your talk. The handouts from a series of weekly talks can serve as a "portfolio" of your work as a student-educator, which could be handed in to the clerkship director at final evaluation time to show the strength of your teaching work.

References

1. Du Q, Sun Y, Ding N, Lu L, Chen Y. Beta-blockers reduced the risk of mortality and exacerbation in patients with COPD: a meta-analysis of observational studies. PLoS One. 2014;9(11):e113048.
2. Wijeysundera DN, Duncan D, Nkonde-Price C, Stangret A, Bachanek M, Trojanowski S, et al. Perioperative beta blockade in noncardiac surgery: a systematic review for the 2014 ACC/AHA guideline on perioperative cardiovascular evaluation and management of patients undergoing noncardiac surgery. Circulation. 2014;130:2246–64.
3. Cornia PB, Packer CD. Perioperative beta-blockade: where do we stand? SGIM Forum. 2015;38(3):5, 14–15
4. Leuppi JD, Schuetz P, Bingisser R, Bodmer M, Briel M, Drescher T, et al. Short-term vs conventional glucocorticoid therapy in acute exacerbations of chronic obstructive pulmonary disease. The REDUCE Randomized Clinical Trial. JAMA. 2013;309(21):2223–31.
5. Poon T, Paris DG, Aitken SL, Patrawalla P, Bondarsky E, Altshuler J. Extended versus short-course corticosteroid taper regimens in the management of chronic obstructive pulmonary disease exacerbations in critically ill patients. J Intensive Care Med. 2017. doi: 10.1177/0885066617741470.
6. Kilic A, Acker MA, Atluri P. Dealing with surgical left ventricular assist device complications. J Thorac Dis. 2015;7(12):2158–64.
7. Lee AYY, Levine MN, Baker RI, Bowden C, Kakkar AK, Prins M, et al. Low-molecular-weight heparin versus a coumarin for the prevention of recurrent venous thromboembolism in patients with cancer. N Engl J Med. 2003;349:146–53.
8. Pitt B, Zannad F, Remme WJ, Cody R, Castaigne A, Perez A, et al. The effect of spironolactone on morbidity and mortality in patients with severe heart failure. N Engl J Med. 1999;341:709–17.
9. Myrick H, Malcolm R, Randall PK, Boyle E, Anton RF, Becker HC, et al. A double-blind trial of gabapentin versus lorazepam in the treatment of alcohol withdrawal. Alcohol Clin Exp Res. 2009;33(9):1582–8.
10. Pedersen JS, Bendtsen F, Møller S. Management of cirrhotic ascites. Ther Adv Chron Dis. 2015;6(3):124–37.

Chapter 14
Future Directions of the Oral Case Presentation

New Technologies at the Bedside

In medicine, recent advances in imaging technology, robotics, pharmacogenomics, phenotypic monitoring, medical informatics, and artificial intelligence have led to big challenges for practicing physicians, who struggle to comprehend the complexities and implications of these new technologies. Third-year medical students, with their shiny new stethoscopes and fresh training in the basic sciences, have been immunized to some degree against future shock by their preclinical studies; they understand many of the new technologies but often struggle to apply them to patients because of their limited knowledge of clinical medicine. As they see more patients and gain experience in the third year, students begin to develop a sense of the big picture, which helps when it comes to evaluating and adopting new technologies.

As clinical medicine and technology converge at the bedside, the student's oral case presentation becomes the crucible where these different elements interact to form something new: an alchemized patient, part flesh and blood, and part genomic data, predictive analytics, and high-tech diagnostic imaging. Instead of a 61-year-old man with newly diagnosed lung cancer, today's new precision medicine patient might be

© Springer Nature Switzerland AG 2019   177
C. D. Packer, *Presenting Your Case*,
https://doi.org/10.1007/978-3-030-13792-2_14

described as "a man with PET CT stage T2aN1M0 EGFR mutation-positive non-small cell lung cancer with high likelihood of response to tyrosine kinase inhibitor therapy" ("O brave new world," as Shakespeare wrote, "that has such people in't").

Over time, the changes wrought by technology will begin to alter the language and format of the oral presentation (Table 14.1). For example, information on the patient's "pharmacogenomic profile" or "relevant mutations" might become an expected part of the write-up and oral presentation, taking its place between the past medical history and family history. Similarly, with the rapid expansion of ultrasound training in US medical schools [1], bedside ultrasound findings will come to be an expected part of the physical exam; in the lung exam, for example, A-lines, B-lines, and lung sliding will be described routinely along with (or perhaps in place of) rales, rhonchi, and egophony. In the assessment and plan, data-mining technologies and artificial intelligence will assist with differential diagnosis and add reliable statistical probabilities to support treatment decisions. The end result will be an invigorated oral presentation with the potential for more diagnostic and predictive power than ever before. This will depend, of course, on how well the student is able to apply the new technologies to the clinical situation at hand. Brilliant answers to the wrong questions will be of no help to a sick patient.

TABLE 14.1 New elements of the oral case presentation

New element	Place in the oral case presentation
"Pharmacogenomic profile" or "relevant mutations"	HPI/PMH/lab results/ assessment and plan
Bedside ultrasound findings	Physical exam
Data-mining technologies and predictive analytics	Assessment and plan
Artificial intelligence	Assessment and plan

Three Ways to Look at an Ambiguous Case

In the following case, a patient with recent onset of shortness of breath and a TIA presents a diagnostic challenge: what is the underlying cause of his dyspnea? Following the case description (below), three hypothetical student assessments are given to illustrate the ways that current and possible future technologies might refocus the oral case presentation:

A 59-year-old African-American man with poorly controlled HTN, type 2 DM, obesity, and a 60 pack-year smoking history presents with 3 days of exertional dyspnea and wheezing. The onset of dyspnea was rapid, over a couple of hours; he has 2-pillow orthopnea but no PND, and he has noticed an increase in his chronic ankle edema over the past week. His weight is up 5 pounds over the past 3 months. No chest pain, palpitations, fevers, chills, sweats, or productive cough; no recent surgery, travel, or immobilization; no personal or family history of venous or arterial thromboembolic disease. He also mentions an episode of right arm and leg weakness with slurred speech 2 days before admission, which resolved completely within 30 minutes; there is no prior history of stroke or similar episodes. Medications are aspirin, lisinopril, HCTZ, metformin, and atorvastatin.

On exam, vital signs are 98.4 96 22 196/112, O_2 saturation 89% on room air. JVP is difficult to assess because of obesity and a short neck but appears to be approximately 8 cm. There is no cervical or intercostal accessory muscle use. Lung auscultation reveals fair air movement and diffuse, moderate expiratory wheezing, with faint bibasilar rales; no rhonchi, egophony, or dullness to percussuion. Heart is regular S4S1S2 with no murmur or rub; abdomen is soft and non-tender, with no masses or organomegaly. In the extremities there is trace-1+ pedal and pretibial edema in both legs to mid-calf. Neurologic exam reveals normal speech with no aphasia, anomia, or dysarthria, normal cranial nerves II-XII, and globally normal motor, sensory, DTRs, and cerebellar exam.

ECG: Normal sinus rhythm at 96/minute; normal P-R interval, no Q-waves, normal QRS and QTc; LVH by voltage criteria with strain pattern in the lateral leads.

Lab results are significant for BUN 22, creatinine 1.3 (baseline 1.1), potassium 3.4, CO2 32, glucose 186, ABG (room air) 7.36/46/68/32/89%, D-dimer 226 (0-500), Pro-BNP 864. Serial troponins are negative.

PA/lateral chest x-ray: Borderline cardiomegaly, possible mild congestion; poor inspiration. No infiltrates or effusions.

Head CT: Chronic microvascular ischemic changes, no acute abnormalities.

Echocardiogram: LVEF 50-55%; grade II diastolic dysfunction; no significant valvular disease; negative bubble study with no evidence of a PFO.

Traditional Assessment and Plan, 2019

This is a 59-year-old man with poorly controlled HTN, type 2 DM, and a 60 pack-year smoking history presenting with 3 days of shortness of breath, wheezing and orthopnea, as well as symptoms consistent with a TIA 2 days ago. On exam, he is hypoxemic and has findings consistent with both mild volume overload and a moderate COPD exacerbation. His echocardiogram reveals diastolic dysfunction, and uncontrolled hypertension is a risk factor for acute decompensated heart failure (ADHF) in patients with diastolic dysfunction. However, his chest x-ray does not clearly show heart failure, his weight gain and leg edema are minimal, and his pro-BNP is in the borderline range for his age group [2]. Orthopnea can occur in COPD as well as in heart failure [3]. Pulmonary embolism is unlikely in view of his Wells score of 0 and normal D-dimer; there is no evidence to support pneumothorax, pneumonia, or acute bronchitis. Regarding the TIA, paroxysmal atrial fibrillation with an embolic episode is a possible etiology that could also explain the abrupt onset of dyspnea and heart failure symptoms.

Since it's not clear whether COPD or ADHF is the primary cause of his dyspnea, we'll treat both conditions with IV diuresis, beta-agonist nebs, and a 5-day course of prednisone with careful monitoring of his volume status. In addition, we'll add amlodipine to his present regimen to improve blood pressure control. For the TIA, we'll prescribe dual antiplatelet therapy with aspirin and clopidogrel indefinitely for secondary stroke prevention [4, 5], order an MRA to evaluate for intra- or extracranial vascular stenosis, monitor for paroxysmal atrial fibrillation on telemetry, and consult neurology for further suggestions.

Technology-Enhanced Assessment and Plan, 2019

This is a 59-year-old man with poorly controlled HTN, type 2 DM, and a 60 pack-year smoking history presenting with 3 days of shortness of breath, wheezing and orthopnea, as well as symptoms consistent with a TIA 2 days ago. On exam, he is hypoxemic and has findings consistent with both mild volume overload and a moderate COPD exacerbation. However, lung ultrasound in our patient reveals multiple B-lines (Fig. 14.1) consistent with pulmonary edema [6], and the lack of respiratory variation in IVC diameter also noted on ultrasound supports a diagnosis of volume overload and ADHF [7]. Based on the normal ejection fraction and findings of diastolic dysfunction on echocardiogram, this appears to be heart failure with preserved ejection fraction (HFpEF), with pulmonary edema likely resulting from uncontrolled hypertension. Regarding the TIA, paroxysmal atrial fibrillation could cause both an embolic TIA and rate-dependent pulmonary edema in a patient with HFpEF. To this point, however, we have not seen evidence of atrial fibrillation on telemetry.

Our plan will be to diurese the patient with IV furosemide, treat the bronchospasm with beta-agonist nebs, and add amlodipine to improve BP control. Since heart failure is the primary problem, we'll hold off on corticosteroids which could aggravate the edema and volume overload. As for antiplatelet treatment for his TIA, there is some evidence to support pharmacogenomic testing for polymorphisms in the CYP2C19 gene that predict poor response to clopidogrel. In a recent Chinese study, the use of clopidogrel plus aspirin compared with aspirin alone reduced the risk of a new stroke

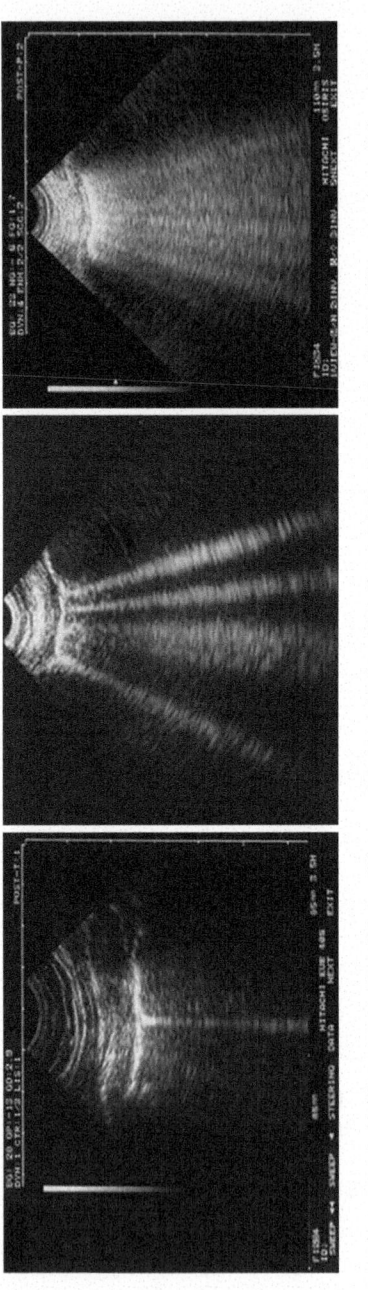

FIGURE 14.1 B-lines. Left: healthy subject, with one isolated B-line, without pathologic significance (possibly minor fissure). Middle and right: pulmonary edema. Several (three or more) B-lines are visible between two ribs, a defining feature of interstitial syndrome. This pattern has been described as "lung rockets." Middle: four or five B-lines are visible. The distance between two B-lines (at the pleural line) is roughly 7 mm in the adult, hence the name "B7-lines." B7-lines correlate with thickened subpleural interlobular septa. Right: seven or eight B-lines are visible, called B3-lines (the distance between two B-lines at the pleural line is roughly 3 mm). B3-lines correlate with subpleural ground-glass lesions. (Reprinted from Lichtenstein et al. [12], Copyright 2009, with permission from Elsevier)

only in the subgroup of patients who were not carriers of the CYP2C19 loss-of-function alleles [8]. I looked into ordering the test – unfortunately, there's a 10-day turnover, and the cost of the test is $379, which will not be covered by the patient's insurance. Also, there are no guidelines at present for CYP2C19 testing in stroke or TIA patients. Given these obstacles, we'll treat with clopidogrel and aspirin according to protocol.

Assessment and Plan for the Same Patient, c. 2029

This is a 59-year-old man with poorly controlled HTN, type 2 DM, and a 60 pack-year smoking history presenting with 3 days of shortness of breath, wheezing and orthopnea, as well as symptoms consistent with a TIA 2 days ago. Based on his history, physical exam findings (including bedside ultrasound with multiple B-lines and lack of IVC respiratory changes), pro-BNP of 864, and a "deep-learning" interpretation of his chest x-ray findings [9] that supports early pulmonary edema, his Watson Database probability of ADHF is 92.4%. A 30-day review of his phonehealth data rules out paroxysmal atrial fibrillation as a potential cause of an embolic TIA and does confirm the timing and duration of his TIA symptoms (38 min) based on speech and motor analysis. Regarding the relevant genomic prescribing data [10], his admission pharmacogenomic panel (see Fig. 14.2, "Future Approach") reveals that he is a poor metabolizer for both CYP2C19 (we will treat with prasugrel rather than clopidogrel for secondary stroke prevention) and CYP2D6 (we will start beta-blocker treatment with a very low dose of carvedilol). He responded well to IV furosemide overnight, and his neurologic status is stable. We'll continue IV diuresis and beta-2 agonist nebs, optimize BP control with the addition of amlodipine and carvedilol, order an MRA to complete the TIA work-up, and initiate our biosensor-based home heart failure care protocol at discharge to optimize

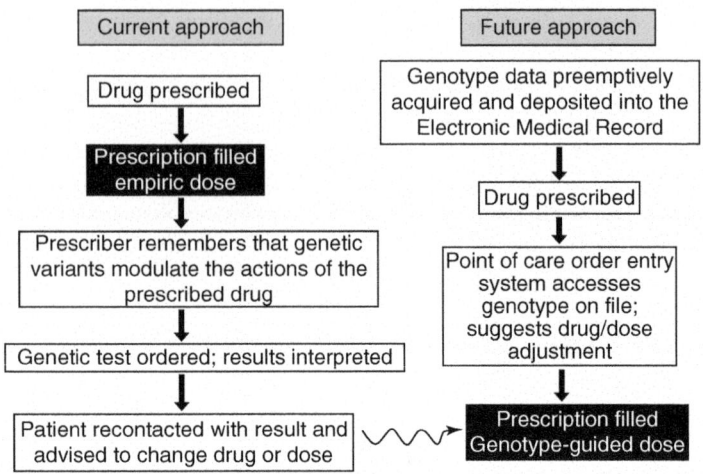

FIGURE 14.2 Contrasting approaches to incorporating genomic information into prescribing. The pathway on the left illustrates current practice, genetic testing on an as-needed basis. The pathway on the right illustrates how preemptive deposit of genotypic data into a genome-enabled electronic medical record would result in rapid and efficient genotype-guided therapy. (Reprinted with permission from Roden et al. [10])

medication adherence, monitor for early signs of decompensation, and prevent rehospitalization [11].

Note the importance of phenotypic monitoring, advanced bedside imaging, data aggregation, artificial intelligence, and "preemptive" pharmacogenomics in the future case presentation. These technologies are in various stages of development and implementation now, but you can be confident that all of them will be fully in play before the close of the next decade. In the meantime, the best way to prepare for the future is to create it yourself: embrace these amazing new technologies, learn to use them, and work to make them better.

References

1. Dinh VA, Fu JY, Lu S, Chiem A, Fox JC, Blaivas M. Integration of ultrasound in medical education at United States medical schools: a national survey of directors' experiences. J Ultrasound Med. 2016;35(2):413–9.
2. Januzzi JL, van Kimmenade R, Lainchbury J, Bayes-Genis A, Ordonez-Llanos J, Santalo-Bel M, et al. NT-proBNP testing for diagnosis and short-term prognosis in acute destabilized heart failure: an international pooled analysis of 1256 patients: the International Collaborative of NT-proBNP Study. Eur Heart J. 2006;27(3):330–7.
3. Dewar M, Curry RW. Chronic obstructive pulmonary disease: diagnostic considerations. Am Fam Physician. 2006;73(4):669–76.
4. Lee M, Saver JL, Hong KS, Rao NM, Wu YL, Ovbiagele B. Antiplatelet regimen for patients with breakthrough strokes while on aspirin: a systematic review and meta-analysis. Stroke. 2017;48(9):2610–3.
5. Johnston SC, Easton JD, Farrant M, Barsan W, Conwit RA, Elm JJ, et al. Clopidogrel and aspirin in acute ischemic stroke and high-risk TIA. N Engl J Med. 2018;379:215–25.
6. Lichtenstein DA, Mezière GA, Lagoueyte JF, Biderman P, Goldstein I, Gepner A. A-lines and B-lines: lung ultrasound as a bedside tool for predicting pulmonary artery occlusion pressure in the critically ill. Chest. 2009;136(4):1014–20.
7. Blehar DJ, Dickman E, Gaspari R. Identification of congestive heart failure via respiratory variation of inferior vena cava diameter. Am J Emerg Med. 2009;27(1):71–5.
8. Wang Y, Zhao X, Lin J, Li H, Johnston SC, Lin Y, et al. Association between CYP2C19 loss-of-function allele status and efficacy of clopidogrel for risk reduction among patients with minor stroke or transient ischemic attack. JAMA. 2016;316(1):70–8.
9. Yasaka K, Abe O. Deep learning and artificial intelligence in radiology: current applications and future directions. PLoS Med. 2018;15(11):e1002707.
10. Roden DM, Wilke RA, Kroemer HK, Stein CM. Pharmacogenomics: the genetics of variable drug responses. Circulation. 2011;123(15):1661–70.

11. Stehlik J, Schmalfuss C, Bozkurt B, et al. Continuous wearable monitoring analytics predict heart failure decompensation: the LINK-HF Multicenter Study. J Am Coll Cardiol. 2018;71(11   Supplement):A646.   https://doi.org/10.1016/S0735-1097(18)31187-2.
12. Lichtenstein DA, Mezière GA, Lagoueyte JF, et al. A-lines and B-lines: lung ultrasound as a bedside tool for predicting pulmonary artery occlusion pressure in the critically ill. Chest. 2009;136(4):1014–20.

Author Index

© Springer Nature Switzerland AG 2019
C. D. Packer, *Presenting Your Case*,
https://doi.org/10.1007/978-3-030-13792-2

Subject Index

Printed and bound by CPI Group (UK) Ltd, Croydon, CR0 4YY
29/04/2026
02099451-0002